Endomor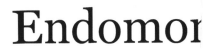

Strategically Use Intermittent Fasting and Flexible Dieting to Work with Your Body Type

Thomas Rohmer

Disclaimer:

This guide has been created for informational and reference purposes only. The author, publisher, and any other affiliated parties cannot be held in any way accountable for any personal injuries or damage allegedly resulting from the information contained herein, or from any misuse of such guidance. Although strict measures have been taken to provide accurate information, the parties involved with the creation and publication of this guide take no responsibility for any issues that may arise from alleged discrepancies contained herein. It is strongly recommended that you consult a physician, personal trainer, and nutritionist prior to commencing this or any other workout or diet plan. This guide is not a substitute for professional personal guidance from a qualified medical professional. If you feel pain or discomfort at any point during exercises contained herein, cease the activity immediately and seek medical guidance.

Before You Begin:

Get the Latest Scoop on the Most Cutting Edge Info on Health & Fitness!

As thanks for picking up this book, I'd love to offer you the chance to maximize your results by getting exclusive info on health and fitness.

You'll be the first to know when I publish new books, and you'll receive exclusive content on health and fitness that I only share with people on my list.

Simply visit the link directly below and get started on the path to the healthiest version of yourself today!

https://rohmerfitness.lpages.co/kindle-sign-up/

Table Of Contents

Introduction

Life gives us challenges, that's for sure. Everyone has his or her ups and downs in life.

Your current struggles might be in regards to your body type. If you're an endomorph, it can almost seem unfair that you were born with such a body type.

It can especially seem this way when you look at other people like ectomorphs, people who can seemingly eat whatever they want and not gain a pound. Sure, you may not have been born with a lightning-fast metabolism like they were, but that doesn't mean all hope is lost.

In fact, being an endomorph isn't all bad; there are actually some advantages to it, contrary to what you might believe. Still, this doesn't take away from the fact that losing weight and keeping it off can be a big-time struggle for endomorphs.

Therefore, specific strategies must be taken in order to achieve lasting results. Regular diet and exercise advice simply won't cut it.

And in this book, I'm going to share with you what you need to be doing differently as an endomorph in order to help you achieve your health and fitness goals.

Also before we get into the nitty gritty of the book please consdier leaving a review if you enjoy it. Even just a few words will help other people know if the book is right for them. Many thanks in advance! Now let's dive in!

Chapter 1: Why the Struggle is Real as an Endomorph

Do you feel like you gain weight just by looking at food sometimes? Almost as if it doesn't matter how little you eat because that food still seems to get stored as body fat?

This is why being an endomorph is a real struggle. Endomorphs have slower metabolisms, which can make it harder for their bodies to burn off the calories from the foods that they eat.

Don't worry though, this book will help you to implement strategies that will help you increase your metabolism over time, and teach you to eat in a way that won't allow your metabolism to destroy any hope you have for success. I'm not saying you'll develop the metabolism of an ectomorph, but improvement is what we're looking to achieve.

There are three main body types—ectomorph, mesomorph, and endomorph. Here's a breakdown of the differences between the three:

Ectomorph: characterized by a smaller bone structure with smaller ankles and wrists. Taller individuals tend to be ectomorphs. They usually have really fast metabolisms and struggle to put on muscle more so than the other two body types.

Mesomorph: a mesomorph is someone in the middle of an ectomorph and endomorph. Most people consider this to be the ideal body type to have because mesomorphs put on muscle easier than ectomorphs, and they don't gain fat as easily as an endomorph does. Metabolism wise, they're right in the middle. Their metabolism isn't nearly as fast as a typical ectomorph, but it's not as slow as an endomorph.

Endomorph: characterized as someone who is stockier and has a larger bone structure—meaning larger ankles and wrists. Endomorphs tend to store fat easily and have lower muscle definition due to the extra adipose tissue. Endomorphic bodies typically use sugar for fuel more so than fat, hence why it can be harder to burn fat. Finally, endomorphs tend to have the slowest metabolism of any of the body types, but building muscle tends to come easier than it does for ectomorphs.

How can I tell if I'm Truly an Endomorph?

Right now you may not totally be sure if you're an endomorph or not. Just because someone is overweight doesn't automatically mean that they're an endomorph.

For example, an ectomorph might suffer from what is commonly referred to as skinny fat syndrome. This is when a person has a low level of muscle mass and also has a higher level of body fat, which makes the stomach stick out.

A person like this would still be classified as an ectomorph who needs to drop the body fat and add some muscle mass in order to solve the problem. With that being said, the easiest way to tell what body type you are is to do the following test—take your thumb and middle finger and wrap them around your opposing wrist.

If your middle finger and thumb don't wrap around fully to touch each other, then you're an endomorph. If you're thumb and middle finger wrap around perfectly to just be touching each other, then you're a mesomorph.

And finally, if your thumb and index finger overlap each other, then you're an ectomorph.

Hopefully, you know now if you're an endomorph or not. And if you are, don't worry.

This book will help give you the strategies that you need in order to succeed. It can be easy to play the blame-game or wonder why you were born a certain way.

However, as you'll see in the coming chapters, wishing to be born with better genetics ultimately won't change anything. Having the right attitude is critical in being able to overcome your weight loss struggles.

Yes, you have more difficult challenges ahead then other people might due to your body type. However, looking at others and comparing yourself to them won't do you the least bit of good.

You have no idea where they're starting from, what they've been through, or what they've done in order for them to get to where they are today. The key here is to focus on yourself and not compare.

I'm going to give you all of the tools you need in order to succeed (not just with diet and exercise but mindset as well), but ultimately, it's still up to you to put these plans into action to get results.

Chapter 2: Why the Game Plan Needs to Change if You Want to See Success

For some people, losing weight comes quite easily. For you though, you might have to work a bit harder at it in order to see success.

What works for one person may not work for you as an endomorph. That's why you're going to need a different game plan from someone else whose body type makes it easier for him or her to get in better shape.

Before we get into the specifics of how things need to change, let's first cover the basic principles of fat loss...

How Does Your Body Burn Fat?

In order to understand the best game plan, it's first important for you to understand how your body actually burns fat. Most people don't know this, but it really isn't that complicated.

Everyday your body has functions that it must maintain, such as breathing and digesting food. These processes require energy in order to continue functioning.

So where do our bodies get the energy it needs in order to continue functioning? It comes from the foods that we eat.

The foods we eat contain energy (i.e. calories), and that energy is then used to help fuel our bodies to move, breathe, and digest food, among many other things. Our bodies only need a certain amount of energy in order to maintain all of these processes.

If you consume more energy than your body needs, the rest will get stored as fat. This is known as a caloric surplus.

On the other hand, if you consume fewer calories than your body needs, it'll tap into your fat stores to get the remaining energy it needs to continuing functioning. This is known as the caloric deficit.

The total amount of energy your body needs in a given day is known as your resting metabolic rate (RMR for short). In other words, your resting metabolic rate is the total amount of calories your body burns off in a given day.

Here's a breakdown of everything I just described:

Mike's resting metabolic rate is 2,300 calories. This means that he burns off 2,300 calories each and every day. Therefore:

- If Mike eats more than 2,300 calories per day, he'll be in a caloric surplus and start to gain weight.
- If Mike eats less than 2,300 calories per day, he'll be in a caloric deficit and start to lose weight.
- If Mike eats right at 2,300 calories per day, he'll be at his maintenance calories and he'll maintain his current bodyweight.

Therefore, if you want to start losing weight you must burn off more calories than you consume. Always remember this!

Every diet that's ever been created has always had the goal of getting you to consume fewer calories in one way or another in order to put you into a caloric deficit. Now some ways are better than others of course.

Most mainstream diets today are set up to make you fail before you even start. And as an endomorph, we need to be strategic with our approach in how we're going to go about creating a caloric deficit.

How Do You Calculate Your Resting Metabolic Rate?

The first step that we need to take is to figure out how many calories it is that you burn off in a given day. The calculation for this is quite simple.

All you need to do is take your current bodyweight and multiply it by 13—that's your RMR. Let's use me as an example:

Current bodyweight=210

210x13=2,730

This means that I burn off 2,730 calories per day. I'll need to start eating less than that if I want to start losing weight.

The question then becomes, how large of a caloric deficit should you create in order to start losing weight? If you create too large of a deficit, you'll be hungry all of the time and eventually crash and burn.

On the flip side, if you create too small of a deficit, then it'll take way too long for you to reach your goal. You want to land somewhere in the middle of these two extremes.

The best way to do that is to aim to lose around one pound of fat per week. At first glance, that might not seem like a lot, er keep in mind that I'm talking about pure fat loss

I'm not talking about losing water weight or anything like that. Losing even 5 pounds of pure fat can make a big difference in how you look.

Imagine one year from now being 52 pounds lighter. It's very possible to do if you go about doing things in the right manner and focus on long-term results rather than quick fixes.

Quick fixes are what most people do when they go on a crash diet to lose 20 pounds in a month. The problem is that these diets are too extreme and people end up going back to their old eating patterns.

And when that happens, so does rebound weight gain. So how much should you eat in order to burn one pound of fat per week?

There are approximately 3,500 calories in one pound of fat (1). This means that you need to create an average weekly caloric deficit of 3,500 calories in order to burn one pound of fat.

Take 3,500 and divide it by 7 days in the week and that comes out to an average daily deficit of 500 calories per day. Let's continue using myself as an example:

Resting metabolic rate: 2,730

2,730-500=2,230

This means that I need to consume 2,230 calories per day in order to start burning off one pound of fat per week.

Remember though, the goal is to create a weekly caloric deficit of 3,500 calories. That means that you could create a larger caloric deficit on some days and a smaller caloric deficit on other days.

For example, if it's a Saturday and you know that you might go out for dinner with your family, you could create a deficit that's smaller than 500 calories. Let's say you create a deficit of 250 calories; this will allow you to enjoy a meal at a restaurant with your family.

Then on a different day, maybe a Tuesday when you don't have much going on, you could create a larger deficit of 750 calories to make up for the smaller deficit. The point is that you can break up things however you please as long as you create an average deficit of 3,500 calories over the course of the week.

If it makes things easier for you to do a 500-calorie deficit every day, then stick with that. However, don't think that you have to create the same sized deficit every day because you certainly don't.

Now that you know how your body burns fat, and you know how many calories you need to eat to start losing weight, let's get into more specifics about what to do diet-wise in order to start burning fat.

Diet Game Plan to Lose Weight as an Endomorph

The body's first source of energy is carbs. Our bodies use carbs for fuel before it taps into our fat stores.

That's true regardless of what body type you are. However, you may have noticed that, as an endomorph, your body may struggle more to burn off carbs, and thus your body is never given the chance to use fat for fuel.

You might have eaten carbs late at night right before bed and then felt like you gained a couple of pounds the next morning. The reason for this is because when we eat food, our insulin levels increase.

Insulin is a hormone that allows glucose from the carbohydrates you eat to enter into cells so that they can be used for energy. The kicker is that the extra glucose will then get converted into lipids and stored as fat for later use.

Not only does insulin signal the body to store fat, but insulin also inhibits the breakdown of fat. This means that your body doesn't burn fat when insulin levels are high.

Essentially, if you're eating a heavy carbohydrate meal right before bed, your body is busy breaking those carbs you just ate down into glucose. Then your body is taking that glucose and putting it into cells and storing the excess as fat instead of burning fat.

This is why one of the strategies we're going to implement is to limit our carbohydrate intake. Notice I said limit, not eliminate.

I want this diet plan to be something that you can do for the rest of your life. If we completely got rid of carbs, then you wouldn't ever be able to enjoy your favorite salty or sugary treats.

Yes, you can still eat foods like chocolate chip cookies and potato chips, and still lose weight if you go about doing it in the right manner, which I'll show you how to do in a later chapter. Carbohydrates aren't the problem in and of itself.

The problem is eating an excessive amount of carbs. Many people act as if carbs are the root of the obesity epidemic, but they're not.

Overeating in general and a lack of exercise is a far more likely cause. Right now though, I want you to understand that if around 50% of your total caloric intake is coming from carbs, than that's too high.

We're going to need to scale that back some so that you can give your body a chance to use fat for fuel instead of carbs. We're going to replace the excess carbs with more protein and fat, which are more satiating than carbs.

This will allow you to stay fuller for a longer period of time while consuming fewer calories overall. This is very important since you're calories are going to be restricted in order to start losing weight.

The next thing we're going to implement is an intermittent fasting protocol. Fasting is essentially where you take a break from eating for a certain period of time.

For example, you might fast for 16 hours of the day and then eat during the remaining 8 hours of the day. I'll explain the exact plan in more detail in the following chapter, but for now, know that the lower carb intake combined with fasting is going to create a powerful fat-burning effect.

I already mentioned why decreasing carb intake is going to be important, but how will fasting help you out? Fasting will define when you can and can't eat.

So for example, if you're fasting for 16 hours a day, you might consume your first meal at noon and your last meal at 8:00 p.m. Then after 8:00 p.m. you'll be fasting for 16 hours until noon again the next day.

This is much better than consuming breakfast soon after you wake up. Breakfast is a lie that we've all been fed from a young age.

We've all been told things such as "breakfast is the most important meal of the day," or "make sure that you eat a big healthy breakfast so you can do well on your test at school today."

Wrong! Wrong! Wrong! Breakfast isn't the most important meal of the day, it's simply a meal, just like any other.

The point of eating is to give our bodies fuel to continue functioning. Therefore, we need to eat when our bodies need fuel.

We don't need to eat because it's a certain time of the day. You're also dehydrated when you first wake up.

Have you ever heard someone tell you that the water you drink at the start of the day is the most important water you'll drink all day? Of course not, that's ridiculous!

You drink water to hydrate your body. It doesn't matter *when* you drink water, what matters is that you hydrate your body when your body is in need of water.

This lie of breakfast has been perpetuated by cereal companies. They needed some way to promote their new breakfast cereals.

And by saying breakfast was the most important meal of the day, they were able to get everyone to buy into this idea that breakfast really was a meal more important than others. On top of that, they would coat their cereals with sugar, preservatives, and other additives to make us hooked on it.

Then we would have to keep coming back for more. Our ancestors didn't eat breakfast.

In fact, they ate more intermittently, similar to what you'll be doing with the fasting plan. They didn't have the luxury of waking up, walking to their fridge, taking out some milk, and then eating a bowl of cereal.

Instead, they had to hunt for their food. Sometimes it would be a while before they found a herd of animals to hunt and feast on.

And if they didn't find any food, they'd of course be fasting in the meantime. So rather than starting your day off with some sugary cereal that's going to spike your insulin and make it harder for you to burn fat, you're instead going to be skipping breakfast.

This will give your body more time to be in a fasted state because you won't be consuming any calories until later on in the day. This'll allow your insulin levels to stay at a low baseline level, giving your body more time to burn fat.

For some people who are looking to lose weight, these strategies may not be necessary. There are plenty of ways to lose weight.

However, as an endomorph, this lower carb and intermittent fasting strategy will help to give you the best chance of success because it works with your body type and not against it.

Chapter 3: The Endomorph Diet Plan

Now it's time for the fun part. We're going to get into the specifics of the diet plan that you need to do in order to start losing weight. I made this into a step-by-step format to make it easy to follow along with:

Step 1: Know How Many Calories It Is That You Need to Eat

We determined this in the previous chapter, but as a quick reminder, take your current bodyweight and multiply it by 13. Then take that number and subtract 500 from it.

For example, if you currently weigh 250 pounds, you would multiply that by 13 and get 3,250. You would then subtract 500 from 3,250 for a total of 2,750.

This is how many calories you need to eat on a daily basis in order to start losing one pound of fat per week.

Step 2: Determine Your Macros

A macronutrient is something your body needs in large quantities in order to sustain life. The three macronutrients are protein, carbs, and fat.

The next step we need to take in our diet plan is to figure out what percentage of our diet protein, carbs, and fat will each consist of. Here's a breakdown of the macro percentages you need to eat:

- Protein - 40%
- Fat - 35%
- Carbs - 25%

You'll notice that's still a fair amount of carbs. It's not a crazy low amount such as 5%, but it's also not high enough to ruin the diet.

This way, you'll still get to enjoy your favorite foods that are carbs. This will help set you up for long-term success instead of quitting and binge eating when the diet gets too hard.

Now we must convert these macro percentages into calories as part of our overall plan. Let's continue using myself as an example.

Recall from earlier that we figured out that I need to consume 2,730 calories per day in order to start losing one pound of fat per week.

Here's how to calculate how much protein, carbs, and fat I need to be consuming based on the percentages from above:

- 2,730x.4=1,092 calories from protein each day
- 2,730x.35=955.5 calories from fat each day
- 2,730x.25=682.5 calories from carbs each day

I can then determine how many grams this equates to by doing the following:

- 1,092/4= 273 grams of protein per day
- 955.5/9= 106.2 grams of fat per day
- 682.5/4= 170.63 grams of carbs per day

Once you've calculated these numbers, it's time to move onto the next step...

Step 3: Track All of the Calories and Macros that You Consume

I'll discuss what to eat in more depth later on, but one of the first things you want to make sure that you're doing is tracking the calories and macros that you eat. You may be surprised to realize just how many calories are in the common foods that we eat.

Most people underestimate how many calories they eat. This causes a big problem—you won't be losing any weight because you're eating more than you think you are!

That's why you must track how many calories it is that you're eating to ensure you're heading in the right direction. Yes, this can be tedious at times, but remember, if you want results that others don't have, you have to be willing to do what others won't do.

And thanks to modern technology, it's not that bad. Simply use your smartphone and download a macro tracking app.

Most of them have similar features and will easily be able to do what you need it for. Once you've downloaded the app, you're simply going to log anything that you eat into the app.

Yes, this also means that you're going to need to log any drinks you consume that contain calories as well. You can type in the foods that you eat into the app, and it'll be able to track how many calories it contains as well as the protein, carb, and fat content.

Most of the apps even have a barcode scanner, which allows you to easily be able to scan the foods you're eating and automatically log the information. One important thing that you'll want to make sure you get right is the portion sizes.

For example, the app obviously won't know how much steak you're eating. That's why it's important to carefully check food labels and measure out your food portions, even using a food scale if necessary.

Sometimes you'll find yourself in a tricky situation. For example, you might be at a restaurant and notice that the nutritional information isn't listed online or on the menu.

If that's the case, you'll want to use the eyeball test in situations such as these. Essentially, you're going to take your best guess as to how many calories are contained within the meal that you're eating.

You'll get better with this as time goes on, so don't sweat too much if you're not sure how many calories something contains. The best rule of thumb to go by when you're guesstimating is to always err on the side of more calories, not less.

This way you won't accidentally overeat and stall your progress. And finally, don't worry about hitting your numbers spot on each and every day.

I'd go nuts if I had to measure and eat exactly 170.63 grams of carbs per day. Get within 5% of the numbers I recommend and you'll be good to go.

Some days, things might work out to where you ate 30% of your total calories from carbs. Other days it might turn out to be 20%. Overall as long as your carbohydrate intake averages out to around 25% or so, you'll be good to go.

Step 4: Implement the Fasting Protocol

Now that you know how many calories, protein, carbs, and fat you need to eat, the next thing you need to do is add in the intermittent fasting protocol. Fasting is going to provide the framework for when to eat.

There are many different styles of intermittent fasting that exist today. Different ones work great for different people.

For example, some people really like to do longer fasts where they might fast for 24-36 hours straight 1-2 times per week. I'm not the biggest fan of these fasting methods for one simple reason—lack of consistency.

Since you're only doing these fasts 1-2 times per week, this can make it harder for your body to get used to fasting. Not only that, but depending on the situation you find yourself in on that day, you might skip the fast all together!

Let's say you do a 36-hour fast starting on Wednesday leading into Thursday. Your friend invites you to dinner to celebrate his birthday that night.

You don't want to turn him down, so you say yes with the caveat that you'll start the fast on Thursday instead. Now you're out of your normal routine and chances are good that you might not even get around to doing that fast.

Imagine if you wanted to try a new sleep schedule where you slept for 11 hours a day 5 days of the week and 30 minutes the other two days of the week. How hard do you think it would be for your body to adapt to that sleeping schedule?

It would be extremely difficult! You could make things much easier on yourself by sleeping a consistent 8 hours each and every night.

That's why I like fasting routines that are more consistent on a day-to-day basis. For example, some fasting protocols have you fasting every day.

This might sound extreme at first, but it's actually way easier to do because you're giving your body a consistent pattern of eating that it can adapt to. And since you're fasting every day, you won't have to fast as long.

Ideally, you'd fast for 16 hours every day; however depending on what your schedule is, fasting for only 14 hours is acceptable as well. Here's a breakdown of what your eating schedule might look like:

- 1st meal of the day: noon
- 2nd meal of the day: 4:00 p.m.
- 3rd meal of the day: 8:00 p.m.

Or

- 1st meal of the day: 1:00 p.m.
- 2nd meal of the day: 5:00 p.m.
- 3rd meal of the day: 9:00 p.m.

The main point is that you want to fast for 16 hours a day, and then have a feeding window of 8 hours. You can start and end your fasts at whatever time you like as long as you're skipping breakfast and not eating for a couple of hours before going to bed.

Also, you don't have to space out each meal equally apart from each other. For example, if eating your second meal of the day at 4:00 is too early, then you could eat your first meal at noon and your second meal at 5:00 when you get off of work.

Then you could eat your third meal at 8:00 or even at a different time. While this is my favorite method of fasting, it's not the only way that you can go about doing things.

There could be special circumstances where you're not going to be able to fast for 14-16 hours in the day. For example, you might be on vacation, and your eating schedule might get thrown out of whack because you're not in control as much for when you're eating.

What should you do in cases like these? You should delay eating your first meal of the day for as long as possible, preferably for at least 5 hours.

For example, if you wake up at 10:00 a.m., then fast for as long as possible after you wake up. Ideally, you'd fast for at least 5 hours until 3:00 p.m.

Since you're on vacation, that might not be possible; if that's the case, simply fast for as long as you can after you wake up. If that means your first meal is at 1:00 and you only fasted for 3 hours after waking, then great.

Yes, this means you're going to have to skip the hotel breakfast, but it'll be worth it. You don't want to use your vacation as an excuse to eat however you please.

You still want to have some sort of plan in place. This way, you'll get the best of both worlds.

You'll still have a fasting plan in place, while at the same time be able to enjoy yourself if you're staying up later than usual eating and drinking. Remember though, this is for special circumstances only.

Most of the time, you're going to aim to fast for 14-16 hours per day and then eat within the 8-hour feeding window. Finally, be sure to check out the frequently asked questions chapter where I cover some common questions about fasting in more depth.

Step 5: Implement and Adjust as Necessary

You now have the foundation you need in order to start your diet plan. What you need to do is finish the rest of this book and then get started as soon as possible.

Nothing will help you learn faster along the way than experience. Start tracking all of your calories and macros.

At first, this won't be the easiest thing to do. However, as time goes on, you'll get better and better at it.

Don't give up on it if it takes a bit of time to get used to. You'll also need to weigh yourself to see if you're making progress or not.

Sadly, most people go about doing this in the wrong way. For instance, they might weigh themselves every day or at different times of the day.

The problem with weighing yourself every day is that our bodyweight fluctuates. The number on the scale is influenced by things such as food in the stomach, or how hydrated you are.

Therefore, if you're weighing yourself every day, you're not getting an accurate measure of if you're truly losing fat or not. Your bodyweight could fluctuate upwards one day and down the next.

Not only that, but imagine what this will do to your psyche. You might step on the scale one day, excited to see that you've lost half a pound.

Then the next day you step on the scale and get disappointed because it shows that you gained a pound. The reality is that you didn't actually gain a pound overnight, your bodyweight is simply fluctuating.

That's why the best thing you can do when it comes to weighing yourself is to weigh yourself periodically enough to account for fluctuations. When you step on the scale, you need to feel confident that it's an accurate reading as to whether you've gained or lost weight.

Weighing yourself once a week will let you know if you're heading in the right direction or not.

In addition, you need to make sure that you weigh yourself at the same time every single time you step on the scale. If you weigh yourself upon waking up one week and in the middle of the afternoon the next, then the reading won't be as consistent.

The best practice is to weigh yourself soon after waking up, right after you go to the bathroom. This way you're weighing yourself on an empty stomach with similar hydration levels every single time.

After tracking your bodyweight for a couple of weeks, you'll want to see if you're making progress or not. If you're losing one pound per week, then great, keep on doing what you're doing.

If you're not losing any weight, or if you're possibly gaining weight, then you need to take a step back and evaluate the situation. The first thing you need to make sure of is that you're accurately tracking your calories and macros.

This is usually where mistakes happen, which can cause you to not get any results. Inaccuracies can happen sometimes because you're not used to correctly measuring portion sizes, and it can take some practice to get good at that.

Other times though, people will feel ashamed to log certain foods that they're eating, or they might cheat and put in smaller portion sizes than they're eating. Remember that no one is going to see your food log expect for you.

You don't have to worry about being judged by anyone. At the end of the day, if you're not doing your best to accurately log what you're eating, then you're only cheating yourself.

This is for your own benefit, so you might as well do it.

The cool thing about tracking all of your calories is that you can see what you've eaten over the past few weeks as well. Look at your food log and see if you notice any commonalities that may have caused you to overeat.

Did you eat too much fast food? Do you eat and drink too much when you're going out with your friends?

By tracking and logging your food intake, patterns will start to appear. Look at certain high-calorie food items that could be holding you back and eat less of them.

See if you've been able to stick to a 14-16 hour fast daily. Are you drinking too much soda or other beverages that contain a high amount of calories?

If so, then these are some areas that you can improve on. The final thing you'll want to consider is if you're adding muscle while dropping fat at the same time.

For example, the number on the scale might not be changing much, and that could be due to the fact that you're replacing the fat you're burning with muscle. If you're lifting weights and want to build muscle, then this isn't a bad thing by any means.

It is something you'll want to be aware of though; you might think that you're not making any progress when, in reality, you are. The last thing you would want to do in a scenario like this is make changes to your diet plan when you don't need to.

If you feel you're adding muscle too quickly, then you could scale back on the weightlifting routine some. Diet wise though, you're doing everything you need to in order to head towards your goals.

Of course, if you think this may be happening to you, then you'll need a way to measure your body fat percentage to make sure that you're heading in the right direction.

As long as your body fat percentage is going down, then you're doing the right thing. The trick is to make sure that you're getting a proper measurement.

One common way people measure their body fat is by using skinfold calipers. These tend to be inaccurate because most people don't have much experience using them.

You have to use the caliper in the same spots in the same exact way for the best accuracy and most people mess it up. If you're going to use skinfold calipers to measure your body fat, make sure you see a professional who has plenty of experience using them.

The best way to get your body fat percentage measured is to use something known as a DEXA scan. This is considered the gold standard for body fat testing in the fitness world.

You'll simply lie down and let the machine scan over you for a couple of minutes. Not only will this tell you what your body fat percentage is, but it'll also measure your muscle mass as well as your bone mass.

The only problem with it is the price. It can cost upwards of 100 dollars or more depending on your location.

Also, it might not be that convenient for you to make appointments to get your body fat tested. This is however, extremely accurate.

If you wanted to, you could get a DEXA scan done at the start of your fitness journey and later on once you've made some considerable progress. If you want a much cheaper option that's easier to use than calipers and can be done in the comfort of your own home, then bioelectrical impedance could be for you.

You can buy it as a handheld device, and it even comes as a feature on some weight scales. It works by sending a small electrical current through your body.

The amount of time it takes for the current to pass through your body will determine what your body fat percentage is. Accuracy wise, this method certainly isn't as good as a DEXA scan.

The readings can vary quite a bit depending on things such as your hydration level, or if you've recently consumed a meal. Dehydration for example, can increase electrical resistance and cause a higher body fat reading.

However, the thing we care about here is consistency. If you're going to use bioelectrical impedance as a way to measure your body fat, then keep things the same every time you use it.

The best way to go about this would be to take your measurement soon after waking up. Similar to how you would weigh yourself first thing in the morning, you could take your body fat reading as well.

Yes, you'll be dehydrated in the morning which will affect the result, but at least you'll have similar levels of dehydration every time you use the device. If on the other hand, you measure your body fat at random times of the day, you might be more hydrated one day than another.

Or the meal you just ate may affect the reading. It may not be the most accurate way to measure your body fat, but it should be able to give you an idea if you're heading in the right direction or not.

And due to the inaccuracies of common ways to measure your body fat, I recommend you only consider regularly measuring your body fat in special circumstances. Namely, this would be if you think you're losing fat and gaining muscle at the same time, causing your overall weight to stay the same.

The weight reading on the scale is going to be the best way to go about things in terms of cost, ease of use, and accuracy, assuming you're weighing yourself in a consistent manner every time.

Also, don't forget that the main thing you want to be concerned with is how you look in the mirror. If you're noticing results with how you look in the mirror, then you know you're on the right track.

However, sometimes it can take a bit of time before you notice significant changes in the way that you look. That's why you want to make sure you have a way of measuring your progress along the way, which is going to be a weight scale in the majority of cases.

Now that we've covered the basic steps you need to take to get your diet plan up and running, let's get into specifics on what you should eat...

What Should I Eat on This Endomorph Diet Plan?

As I've talked about before, the big problem with a lot of mainstream diets is that they tell you what you can and can't eat. One diet might say that you can never eat anything with sugar in it ever again.

Yes, I agree that not eating sugar is a very healthy thing to do. However, is it realistic to think that someone could go the rest of his or her life without consuming sugar ever again?

Sure there's going to be that rare case, but it's few and far between. Most people would fail on such a diet plan because we are biologically hardwired to seek out sugary and salty foods due to their richness in calories.

No, this isn't an excuse to eat these types of foods all of the time. Instead, it's wiser to limit sugar intake, but not get rid of it altogether.

This way you'll still be able to enjoy your favorite foods that contain sugar from time to time, such as brownies or cake. And it's because of unsustainable diet plans such as no sugar diets that cause people to get caught in the vicious yo-yo dieting cycle.

They'll put themselves through misery to lose weight, only to quit when they can't take it anymore and then slowly start to gain all of the weight back. That's why I'm not going to tell you specifically what you can and cannot eat.

I want this to be a long-term approach where you're able to lose weight and keep it off for good. That's why I'm instead going to give you guidelines for what kinds of foods you should eat, and then you can fill in the rest.

If I told you what to eat for every single meal, that would be like you riding a bike using training wheels. The training wheels are the only thing that allow you to be able to successfully ride the bike.

What would happen if you were in a situation where you couldn't eat what I told you to? The training wheels would be taken away and you'd struggle to ride the bike.

This approach will make you much better off for long-term success because you'll be more in tune with your own body.

Follow My Golden 85% Rule

When it comes to eating your favorite foods versus healthy foods, how do you go about striking a balance? Eating junk food all of the time will make it extremely difficult to keep your overall calories low.

Not only that, but you'll be dealing with a lot of food cravings thanks to the blood sugar crashes. Eating healthy all of the time can lead to burnout, causing you to binge eat and feel guilty about yourself.

That's why you should eat healthy foods 85% of the time and the remaining 15% of the time eat foods you enjoy. This allows you to strike the perfect balance between clean foods and junk food.

Remember it's not what you eat 15% of the time that causes obesity problems—it's what you eat the majority of the time that causes problems. What exactly constitutes something as healthy though?

My general rule is to think of our ancestors. If it wasn't possible for them to eat something back in the day, then it should be part of the 15%.

You want to consume foods that contain as few of ingredients as possible. Now, this isn't a hard and fast rule.

For example, let's say you're going to have pasta for dinner one night. If you're worried about whether or not white pasta should go in the 15% category, then you're overthinking things.

Put it in the 85% and move on. Generally, you know what's good and what's not.

Sugary desserts and salty snacks like potato chips go in the 15% category. These are foods that you want to enjoy from time to time.

Things like vegetables and lean meats should go into the 85% category. Here's a non-comprehensive list of some healthy foods you could eat as part of your diet plan:

- Fruits
- Vegetables
- Sweet potatoes
- Brown Rice
- Avocados
- Various types of nuts and seeds
- Different kinds of beans
- Quinoa
- Cottage cheese
- Coconut oil

You might also be wondering how you know if you're eating a proper ratio of healthy to unhealthy foods. Well just like with the macros, it's doesn't have to be spot on.

Just try to get around those numbers. Over the course of a week, it should average out to roughly 85% healthy foods and 15% not so healthy foods.

You can take these percentages and factor them into your total caloric intake. For example, if I'm eating 2,230 calories per day, then approximately 335 of those calories can come from junk food.

The remaining 1,895 should come from clean sources. In this example, 335 calories per day might not seem like a lot, but remember you can divide it up how you like.

You could eat all 335 calories every single day, which would maybe mean eating a small bowl of ice cream or some potato chips. Or you could save up those calories and use them for later.

For instance, you could go three days eating only healthy foods, which would allow you to eat a meal consisting of 1,005 calories of whatever you wanted. Finally, you could even save up all of your junk calories for one day of the week where you can essentially have a cheat day.

The choice is yours. You do want to make sure that you're still properly counting and tracking your macros.

To be clear, these aren't extra calories that you're adding into your diet plan. You're still going to eat the same amount of calories and macros that we calculated earlier.

Let's say for instance you eat some candy that contains 30 grams of carbs. You still need to factor that in towards your 25% total daily carbohydrates that you're going to be eating for the day.

Chapter 4: Why Me? The Correct Endomorph Mindset You Need to Have

Having the correct mindset is something that most people struggle with when it comes to achieving their health and fitness goals. However, as an endomorph, it's especially critical that you have the proper mindset to ensure success with your health and fitness goals.

The main reason for this is because it can be easy to compare yourself to people who are naturally slender, and wonder why you couldn't have been born with a metabolism like theirs. This mindset is what can then hold you back from taking the action necessary in order to reach your goals.

If you don't think that diet or exercise will work for you, then you won't take the necessary action and you'll stay stuck.

That's why it's so important to make sure you have the proper mentality to realize that it is possible for you to be able to achieve your goals, regardless of how many times you've failed in the past, or if you've been overweight your whole life. None of that matters.

All that matters is the present moment and where you're going from this day forward. That's the first thing I need you to do—let go of anything from your past that might be holding you back.

Forgive yourself and move forward. You owe it to your future self. I know how bad it can be to hold onto failures from the past.

For instance, I have many regrets from my senior season of high school basketball. My team didn't achieve the goals that I had in mind for the season, and as the leader of the team, I felt like I let a lot of people down—especially myself.

In fact, I still have dreams about my senior season to this very day. I'm telling you from my own personal experience that you have to let the past be the past, even if it's really hard.

You have to use it as a learning experience. For instance, this whole experience has taught me that I have to do everything in my power to achieve a certain outcome that I want.

I can't leave anything on the table because if I do, then I might end up with the same regret that I did back when I was in high school. The best way that I've been able to help myself move on from this was to forgive myself.

I didn't have all the knowledge back then that I have now. In fact, I wouldn't be where I am today if it weren't for my past failures and mistakes.

I'm sure the same can be said for you. Maybe you've tried dieting and exercising in the past and it didn't work for you.

It's okay if that's the case. Simply forgive yourself because you probably didn't have the right information.

Back then, you didn't know everything that you're learning in this book. So use your past failures as learning experiences.

At least now you know some things that didn't work for you. That's great!

You don't have to worry about wasting your time on those things in the future. Forgiveness and permission to be imperfect are the best ways to move on from the past.

The reality is that even with the right information, there will still be times when you slip up or make mistakes, which leads me to my next tip...

How You Should Handle Setbacks

Even if you have moved on from the past, the reality is that mistakes you make in the present can trip you up too. These mistakes will then become a recent memory in your past, which can then hold you back in the future.

That's why when a mistake does happen and you fall down, you must get back up immediately and keep on moving forward as if nothing happened. That's the best way to handle setbacks.

The more you sit there and dwell and worry about your mistake, the more it'll keep popping up in your mind to try and sabotage you. You have to remember that work beats worry.

If you get right back up and keep on working towards your goal, that depressing thought will lose its power and go away. It's easy to see how mistakes made along the way could trip up even the most enthusiastic of individuals.

You make a mistake, and then you start to wonder why you did that. Then thinking of that thought makes you think about it even more.

Then the mistake will start to paralyze you from taking any action in the future. And once the action stops, so do the results that you're getting.

Therefore, the best thing you can do is always be laser-focused on moving forward. Get that tunnel vision and move forward at all costs.

Another thing you can do to help yourself with this is to remind yourself that you're imperfect. If you try to be perfect and then fail, your mind won't hesitate to let you know that you did an action that's inconsistent with the perfect person you're supposed to be.

However, if you embrace your imperfections instead, then you're essentially telling yourself that you're human and you make mistakes from time to time. Then when a mistake does happen, it's not the end of the world.

You'll find that it will be much easier to move on from it.

Why You Shouldn't Compare Yourself to Others

A point I briefly mentioned earlier is that you shouldn't compare yourself to others. Doing so will only make you feel worse about yourself and wonder why it is that you have to go through the struggles that you do while others don't.

Playing the comparison game is one that you'll never be able to win. So if you regularly notice that you compare yourself to others, what are some things that you can do?

The first thing I want you to take a look at is your social media use. There is research to show that there is a correlation between social media usage and depression (2). That is to say that the more time you spend on social media, the more likely it is that you're going to have some degree of depression.

Why is that? Well think about what it is that you see when you log onto any of the popular social media sites—you see all sorts of amazing and exciting things!

This person bought a new house, so and so got a new promotion, a friend from high school just got engaged, somebody had a kid, somebody else just had a killer workout and on and on it goes. Social media is a highlight of people's lives.

And that makes total sense. People are only going to share the best and most exciting things that are happening in their lives in order to generate the most likes.

And when you constantly see these things, it's going to make you feel like you're not adequate. You're going to wonder why you're struggling to get fit while everyone else is living their dream life with fulfilling work, relationships, and travel to cool places.

The reality is that a lot of social media is an exaggerated truth. People will make their lives seem better than they actually are in order to get more attention on social media.

The game of seeing what posts or pictures can generate the most likes is a never-ending cycle. The fact of the matter is that a lot of our lives consist of boring and mundane things— driving to work, eating, sleeping, watching t.v., etc.

Rarely do exciting things happen. Yet when you're friends with 500 people on social media, it can sure make it seem as if something new and exciting is happening all of the time.

Guess what though? It's not!

That's why the best thing you can do is limit or eliminate entirely the use of social media. This will help you not compare yourself to others as much.

I noticed big leaps in my happiness once I stopped using social media. Of course, if you want to use it to connect with an old friend and actually meet up to hang out with him or her in person, then go for it.

For the most part though, you're definitely better off not using it and instead focusing on what it is that you need to do in order to reach your goals.

If you're able to limit or stop using social media altogether, then congratulations! You've taken a major step towards not comparing yourself to others. You won't know how good it'll be for you until you try, so definitely give it a shot!

However, that's not the only thing that you need to do. There's still a lot of other stimulation we receive every day from advertisements.

These ads are designed to make us want to desire a certain thing. It might be a "flawless" model trying to sell us makeup for example.

And if only we had this thing, then it would finally be the key we need to unlock our happiness. Of course, that's rarely the case.

Therefore you also need to limit the stimulation you receive from ads. This isn't the easiest thing to do.

No matter what, you're not going to be able to stop seeing all ads unless you decide to live under a rock. Even with that being the case, there are still some practical things you can do to help limit the use of ad stimulation.

You might be wondering how all of this ties into losing weight as an endomorph, but trust me, all of these things affect our mindset and our moods, which in turn determines our actions, which determines our results. Mindset really could be the thing that's been holding you back, so please give this advice a shot before you immediately dismiss it.

Number #1: Limit use of the radio

When you're driving your car to work, the grocery store, or wherever else, I want you to consider doing something besides listening to the radio. The reason for this is not just to avoid the ads, but also because of the songs that you'll be listening to.

What are most songs today about? Usually, it's about love or getting money depending on the genre of the song.

And if you're single or broke, this can really make you feel depressed. You might think that the reason why you're single is that you're struggling to get fit.

I'm not saying that you should never listen to the radio or music in general ever again. What I want you to do is to start paying attention to how you feel after listening to mainstream music on the radio.

Then give up the radio for a couple of weeks and see how you feel. Notice how you feel after listening to certain genres, maybe you need to listen to different kinds of music.

The reality is that music can negatively or positively affect our moods and our thoughts—as some research indicates (3). Therefore you need to be more conscious of the kind of music that you do listen to in order to ensure that music isn't subconsciously affecting your mood in a negative way.

And finally, if you're not sure of what else to do in your car if you're not going to listen to music, then consider listening to podcasts, audiobooks, or just have complete silence. There's nothing wrong with some quiet time every now and then!

Number #2: Be smart about watching television

The next big way most of us see ads is during breaks on the television shows we watch. Again the more ads we're exposed to, the more likely it is to negatively affect our mindset and thus our ability to get results.

Therefore it's wise to limit the use of, if not stop watching t.v. altogether. You may not want to stop watching t.v. altogether and if so that's okay.

But you do need to be more conscious about how you're consuming it. For instance, you could pre-record your shows and then watch them later.

This will allow you to be able to fast forward through the ads when they come on. You could also watch your shows using an online subscription service that doesn't contain any ads.

Number #3: Use an ad blocker when you're on the internet

The final thing you can do to limit the number of ads that you see is to use an ad blocker on your internet browser. This will block ads that you'd normally see when you're browsing through articles on the internet.

Again every little bit helps, so try this out and see what kind of a difference it makes.

The Correct Way to Set Goals to Increase Your Chances of Success

Most of the world doesn't set goals. Most people don't really know what it is that they want, or they have a vague idea of what they want to achieve.

Imagine being an archer but not having a target to aim and shoot at. It's impossible to win!

On the contrary, imagine having a laser focus on the target you're trying to shoot. Nothing else is distracting you from hitting the bull's eye.

By setting goals, you'll be able to focus in on what it is that you truly want. Things won't be able to easily distract you anymore.

Setting goals will make what you want real; if used right, they'll also create a sense of urgency that will encourage you to take the necessary action in order to accomplish your goals. Here's the wrong way to go about setting a goal:

- I want to lose weight.

This is nothing more than a vague idea in your head. If it happens then great, but no big deal if it doesn't.

It's as if your goal is in a bottle in the middle of the ocean and you're hoping it'll magically find its way to the correct destination. Here's a much more powerful way to set your goals:

- I lose 10 pounds of fat by January 31, 2019.

So what is it that makes writing your goals in this manner so much more effective? Well, the first thing is that you need to write it down physically with pen and paper.

This makes your goal real and not an idea in your head. Ideally, you would write your goal down first thing in the morning and before you go to bed each night.

This way it'll be what you think about when you first wake up and the last thing you think about before you go to bed. Secondly, the goal is written in the present tense as if it's already been achieved.

This has a much more powerful effect on the subconscious than saying something like 'I will lose 10 pounds of fat'. The reason is that it makes your mind think that you've already achieved the goal.

Your subconscious mind doesn't know the difference between something that's real versus something that's being vividly imagined. Therefore, we can take advantage of this by acting as if we've already achieved our goal, and imagining what it would look and feel like to have accomplished this goal.

This goal is also specific. It targets a certain amount of weight to be lost.

Instead of generally saying you want to lose weight, you have a specific number in mind. Not only that, but what kind of weight do you want to lose? Muscle mass? Water weight?

I'm assuming what you want to lose is fat. That's why the goal says to lose 10 pounds of *fat*.

This gives us a specific target to aim for. The final thing you'll notice about this goal is that there's a deadline attached to it.

If you don't put a deadline to your goals, then it's as if you're saying to yourself, "I'll get around to achieving this when I have the extra time." And you and I know good and well that time will likely never come.

That's why you must set a deadline for when you'll achieve your goal. Remember there's no such thing as an unrealistic goal, just unrealistic time frames.

If your deadline ends up being too ambitious and you don't reach your goal by then, don't sweat it. You can always set a new deadline for when you'll achieve the goal by.

The main thing is that you don't skip this creating a deadline. A deadline will help create the urgency necessary in order for you to be able to get the job done in a timely manner.

Find Your Why

After you set a goal for what it is that you want to achieve, the next thing that you need to do is find your why. Finding your why is a powerful motivator that can help drive you to achieve your goal.

Similar with setting goals, there's a right and a wrong way to go about doing this. If you have an idea as to why you want to achieve something in your head, that likely isn't strong enough for you to be able to get the job done.

Just like with writing your goals down, you also need to write your reason why down. Not only that, most people only scratch the surface when it comes to finding their why.

Someone might say for example that he or she wants to get healthy. However, that might only be a surface reason for what the person truly wants.

You must dive deeper. The best way to do that is to ask yourself why three times. For example:

Why do you want to lose weight?

I want to look and feel better about myself.

Why do you want to look and feel better about yourself?

So I can go out on more dates.

Why do you want to go out on more dates?

So I can be in a relationship.

45

Therefore, the main thing that would be driving this person would be so that he or she can be in a relationship. If he or she stopped with "I want to look and feel better about myself", then he or she likely wouldn't be motivated to keep on moving forward.

That reason wouldn't be compelling enough. However, now that we got to the root of what it is that the person truly wants, this can be a much more powerful motivator.

At the end of the day, we're all driven by something, so you might as well find out what it is that you truly want and then go for it. Think about it in this way—why do some people stick around at a job they hate for years on end?

Asking why can help us get to the bottom of that:

Why do I work at a job that I loathe?

So I can pay for my bills.

Why do I want to pay my bills?

So I can afford to eat and have a roof over my head.

Why do I want to eat and have a roof over my head?

Because starving and not having a place to live would be worse than going back to my job.

So in the end, staying at a job someone hates is easier and better than not being able to eat or have a place to live. Staying at a job you hate can also be easier than updating your resume, applying for a new job, interviewing, hoping you get the job, and then learning the ins and outs of the new job.

When you think of all that you have to do in order to get a new job, it can be much easier to stay put where you're at. That's why, when it comes to weight loss or any other endeavor worth achieving, you must focus on the next step and nothing else.

For example, when you think about all that you have to do in order to workout at the gym—change into workout clothes, drive to the gym, workout, come home, and shower, it can be quite daunting.

However, if you only think about the next step, then things won't seem as bad. If you told yourself all I'm going to do is change into gym clothes, then that's a lot less intimidating than the thought of everything else you'll have to do.

Then once your gym clothes are on, ask yourself what the next step is and do that. Before you know it, you'll have completed the entire process of going to the gym without it feeling like such a big chore.

To think of it in another way, imagine your life like an hourglass. In an hourglass, only one grain of sand can pass through at a time. Yes, sand is continuously passing through the hourglass, but it still is coming through one grain at a time.

Much is the same in our lives. Time is continually passing us by regardless of what we do.

Even with that being the case, there's still only one thing we can do before we move onto the next thing. For example, you don't change your clothes and appear at the gym to workout all at once.

You change your clothes, then you drive to the gym, and then you workout. Breaking your tasks up into smaller chunks makes it far easier to consume and makes it more likely that you'll actually do it.

And speaking of things you need to do in order to achieve your goals, let's not forget about process goals...

Don't Forget About Process Goals

There are outcome goals and process goals. The type of goal we talked about earlier is an outcome goal.

Process goals are what you have to do in order to achieve your outcome goals. It helps if you think of this as a mountain—the outcome goal is like the top of a mountain; it's where you want to go.

Process goals are what you must do in order to reach the top of the mountain. Here's an example:

Outcome goal: I lose 10 pounds of fat by January 31, 2019.

Process goal: I workout 3 days per week at 7:00 a.m. Monday, Wednesday, and Friday.

Having a desired outcome is great, but that won't do you much good if you don't have a game plan laid out for what it is that you need to do in order to achieve that outcome goal.

And when I'm talking about a plan, I'm talking about a specific one. Notice how the process goal wasn't something vague like, "I workout 3 days per week."

It needs to be more specific than that. What time are you going to workout at? What days of the week, etc.?

Make sure you have a plan in place for each process goal. This will make it all the more likely that you'll actually do what you need to do.

Remember that failing to prepare is setting yourself up for failure, and having vague process goals is telling yourself that it's not that important.

The final question then becomes, how many process goals should you have? Working out 3 days per week is great, but that may not be the only thing you need to do in order to reach your goal.

That's why I recommend that you have 3 process goals with every one outcome goal that you have. Think to yourself about what the 3 main things are that you need to do in order to be successful.

In the case of losing 10 pounds of fat, it could be something like:

1. Exercising a certain amount.
2. Eating a certain number of meals that consist of healthy food choices.
3. Getting the proper amount of sleep.

Of course, saying you'll get the proper amount of sleep or making healthy food choices isn't specific enough. Everyone knows that they need to do that, and yet most people struggle to do these things on a regular basis.

Here's a better way to make them more specific:

- I eat three meals per day at noon, 4:00 p.m. and 8:00 p.m. My meals consist of wholesome food choices that are high in protein, moderate in fat, and low in carbs.
- I sleep for 8 hours each and every night. I go to bed at 11:00 p.m. and wake up at 7:00 a.m. 7 days per week.

Hopefully, you can notice a difference in making your process goals specific. Now you have a much better game plan moving forward as to what it is you need to do in order to achieve your outcome goal.

Are you enjoying this book so far? If so, please consdier leaving a review. Even just a few words would help others decide if the book is right for them!

Chapter 5: Endomorph Exercise—How to Workout in a Way That's Optimal for Your Body Type

Make no mistake about it—you don't *have* to exercise in order to achieve your weight loss goals. However, it'll make things much easier on yourself, especially as an endomorph.

Think of exercise as a bonus; it'll either give you some more leeway in your nutrition plan, or it'll help you reach your goal that much faster. The reason why I say that you don't have to exercise in order to get results is that you can lose weight by focusing solely on your nutrition plan.

If your diet plan is solid, then that alone could be enough to get you to where you want to go. The reality is that you can't out-exercise a bad diet.

So for example, you could eat a burger, fries, and milkshake at a fast food restaurant. That meal could easily contain at least 2,000 calories.

Needless to say, it would take a very very long time in order for you to burn off the equivalent to that. You would almost have to run the equivalent of a marathon in order to fully burn off that meal.

That's not a fair deal. The better way to go about things is to not eat that meal in the first place.

That way any exercise you do can be seen as a bonus instead of a desperate attempt to make up for something you shouldn't have eaten.

What Kind of Exercise Should You Do?

One of the characteristics of an endomorph is that they're the strongest and contain the most muscle mass of the 3 different body types. With that being the case, it makes sense to do exercise routines that are based on those strengths.

Doing something like long and boring cardio probably isn't the best option for endomorphs. It's a common myth that doing cardio is the best way to burn fat.

The reality is that exercise burns calories, and burning calories will help to put you into a caloric deficit, which is how your body will burn fat. Therefore, you shouldn't worry as much about the type of exercise that you're doing.

Instead, focus on what your strengths are and what you enjoy doing. That's what you'll stick to in the long run.

It doesn't matter how good an exercise plan is, if you quit and give up on it, then it won't work. That's why I want you to do something that's more fun than jogging on a treadmill.

Not only that, but you might as well exercise in a way that's optimal for your body type. So what type of exercise should you do?

Well if you shouldn't do slow cardio, then you should do the opposite. The opposite of slow is high intensity and the opposite of running is resistance training.

Therefore the type of exercise that's best for an endomorph is high-intensity resistance training.

Why High-Intensity Workouts are Best for Endomorphs

So what is it exactly that makes high-intensity workouts so great for endomorphs? Well consider this—endomorphs have the slowest metabolisms of the 3 different body types.

Therefore, endomorphs need to do workouts that will help to increase their metabolisms. You're definitely not going to have that happen by doing slow cardio.

However, if you lift as heavy as possible and keep the rest periods short, this will keep your heart rate up, and as a result, help to boost your metabolism. Not only that, but an endomorph's body was designed to workout in this type of manner.

It was made to do high-intensity work for short periods of time. An ectomorph was made to do something more along the lines of long-distance work such as a marathon.

You'll probably enjoy doing these types of workouts more than going on a 5-mile run for example.

Endomorph Workout

The ideal endomorph workout is one where you're first and foremost training with mostly compound exercises. A compound exercise is one that works on multiple muscle groups at the same time.

An example of this would be the barbell squat. The squat primarily works on the quads, hamstrings, and glutes.

On the other hand, an isolation exercise primarily works on one muscle group at a time. An example of an isolation exercise is something like a leg extension.

The leg extension only works on the quads. Filling your workout routine with a bunch of isolation exercises would be a waste of your time in the sense that you won't be doing things as efficiently and effectively as you could be.

After that, you want to make sure that you're training with higher rep ranges—around 12-15 reps per set. A rep is a single completion of an exercise.

On the squat for example, you would squat down and then stand back up. That would be one rep of the exercise.

A set is a series of reps. For example, if you were doing 3 sets of 12 reps on squat, you would squat down and then come back up completing one rep of the exercise.

You would do that 11 more times and that would complete 1 set of the exercise. You would then take a rest period (in this case let's say one minute) and once the rest period is over you would complete another 12 reps for set number 2, rest again for one minute and then complete set number 3 by doing another 12 reps.

Once all 3 sets of 12 reps have been completed, you would then move onto the next exercise in the workout routine. The reason why we want to do higher reps here is that this is going to help to keep the heart rate up.

It'll help to keep the intensity of the workout high and allow you to burn more calories overall. Don't get me wrong, training in lower rep ranges and taking longer rest periods certainly has its place, especially if you're a powerlifter or something along those lines.

However, for the average endomorph who's looking to optimize his or her time in the gym to maximize fat-burn, this is going to be the best way to go about doing things. Speaking of rest periods, you'll want to rest for 30-60 seconds in between sets for your exercises.

This again will help to keep your heart rate up and make sure that the workout stays intense. If you take 3-5 minutes of rest in between sets, then that's enough time for your heart rate to come down some.

The final thing you need to consider is how heavy of a weight you should use. A good rule to follow is that you always want to lift as heavy of a weight as possible for the given rep range.

So if you were completing 5 reps of an exercise, you're going to use more weight than if you were doing 15 reps for the same exercise. However, that doesn't mean you should use so light of a weight that the 15 reps isn't challenging.

You want the last 1-2 reps of the exercise to be extremely challenging. In fact, it's better to pick a weight that's too heavy and causes you to fail at rep number 13 out of 15 than it is to pick a weight that's too light and stop at 15 when you could've done more.

It comes down to having the right mentality. If the workout says to get 15 reps and we're not sure how much weight to use, we tend to err on the side of a weight that's too light.

Even though we could push ourselves past 15 reps, we stop at 15 because that's what our workout told us to do. You might not know how much weight you should be using if it's your first time doing an exercise, so at that point take your best guess.

If you're able to easily get 15 reps without any sort of challenge, then increase the weight for the next set. Keep adjusting the weight as necessary until you get to the point where the last 1-2 reps are very challenging.

And over time, you want to make sure that you're increasing the amount of weight that you're lifting. If you lift the same weight with the same exercises and the same reps, your body will catch on to what you're doing and progress will stall.

Therefore, whenever you can successfully complete all of the reps for a given exercise, increase the weight the next time you do the exercise. Let's use an example of doing 3 sets of 15 reps of the dumbbell military press exercise:

Workout #1: Weight being used — 30-pound dumbbells

- Set 1:15 reps
- Set 2:13 reps
- Set 3: 12 reps

Since the lifter wasn't able to complete 15 reps on sets 2 and 3 he should stick with the 30-pound dumbbells until he can do 15 reps on all 3 sets. Let's say on his next workout he is able to complete 15 reps on all 3 sets using the 30-pound dumbbells.

That's great, and for the next workout he should increase the weight to the next set of heavier dumbbells. In most gyms, this will likely mean using 35-pound dumbbells.

And if on his first time using 35-pound dumbbells he's unable to hit 15 reps per set that's okay. He'll stick with that same weight until he's able to do 15 reps for all 3 sets and then increase the weight once again.

This is a principle known as progressive overload, which states that you always need to be challenging your body in order for it to keep on growing. That's why with each and every workout you want to try and increase the number of reps you're doing or the amount of weight that you lift.

For example, let's say that you're aiming to complete 12 reps of an exercise. The first time you do it, you get 12 reps on the first set, 11 on the second, and 9 on the third set.

The next time you do that exercise, strive to do more reps on your second and third sets. You still might not hit 12 reps on all 3 sets, but maybe you'll be able to do 12 on the first, 12 on the second, and 11 on the third.

That's great because you're still making process and giving your body a challenge. You would still stick with that weight until you're able to do 12 reps on all 3 sets before increasing the weight.

Here's a sample full body workout that you can do in the gym 2-3 days per week:

- Dumbbell Squats: 3 sets of 12 reps, 60 seconds rest between sets
- Dumbbell Bench Press: 3 sets of 12 reps, 60 seconds rest between sets
- Lat Pulldowns: 3 sets of 12 reps, 60 seconds rest between sets
- Standing Dumbbell Military Press: 3 sets of 15 reps, 45 seconds rest between sets
- Standing Dumbbell Curls: 3 sets of 15 reps, 30 seconds rest between sets
- Tricep Pushdowns: 3 sets of 15 reps, 30 seconds rest between sets

Don't let the simplicity of this workout fool you. Often times it's the simplest things that are the most effective.

Doing this workout 2-3 times per week will give you some great benefits. Many people sadly think that full body workouts are a waste of time and instead prefer a bro-splits routine, where you only workout one muscle group per session.

Full body workouts are going to be awesome for you as an endomorph for the following reasons:

- You'll burn more calories in less time thanks to the metabolically demanding compound exercises.
- You'll experience a better recovery of your nervous system because you won't be lifting weights on consecutive days.
- You'll be able to gain strength and build muscle faster since you're working out your major muscle groups multiple times per week.
- And if you're new to weight training, you'll master the exercises sooner because you'll be performing them more often.

Make sure you have at least one day of rest in between each workout. For example, if you're working out 3 days per week you could workout on a Monday, Wednesday, and Friday.

Should I Not Waste My Time Doing Cardio as an Endomorph?

It's not that you shouldn't do any cardio as an endomorph. Cardio can still give you some good results if you do it in the right way.

Doing cardio in the wrong way is a waste of your time because you're not doing things as efficiently as you could be. That's why I want to share with you the most effective way to do cardio.

The reason why I say this is because it allows you to burn the most amount of calories in the least amount of time. Here's the first part of the cardio workout:

High-intensity interval training

High-intensity interval training (HIIT for short) is essentially where you alternate between a period of high-intensity exercise and a period of low-intensity exercise. For example, if you were doing a HIIT workout on a treadmill, you might alternate between running at a speed of 7mph and walking at a speed of 3 mph.

This is way better than doing something like jogging. The reason is that this type of intense workout fits perfectly with the endomorph body type.

HIIT will do a better job of helping you reach your max heart rate. It'll do a better job of boosting your metabolism compared to slow and steady state cardio.

Now you can do HIIT on any cardio machine of your choice whether that be that a treadmill, an elliptical, a stairmaster, a rowing machine, or even on an outdoor track. Whatever you choose doesn't matter.

What does matter is that you alternate between a high-intensity and a low-intensity. Let's say for example, you're doing your HIIT workout on a treadmill.

How fast should you run for during the high-intensity part and at what pace should you go for the low-intensity part? Basically, for the high-intensity part of the workout, I recommend going at a pace where you would be pushing yourself.

Not so much to the point where you might pass out, but to where it's a challenge. That will be different speeds for different people.

For some people that might mean running at 10 mph, for others 7 mph, or maybe 6 mph. Your high-intensity speed will also depend on the duration of the intense exercise.

For example, there are many different high-intensity to low-intensity ratios you can do. You could run for a minute and walk for a minute.

You could do 30 seconds of running and 1 minute of walking. You might also do 1 minute of running and 2 minutes of walking.

The point is to adjust things based on your current fitness level. Ideally, you'd work your way up to a 1:1 ratio where you're running for the same length of time that you're walking.

Initially though, you might not be at that point. And thanks to the efficiency of this workout, you can burn quite a few calories in a short period of time such as 15 minutes. Here's an example HIIT workout you could do on a treadmill:

High-Intensity Exercise for 30 seconds consisting of running on a treadmill at 7 mph.

Alternated with:

Low-Intensity Exercise for 1 minute consisting of walking on a treadmill at 3 mph.

Repeat for a total of 10 rounds until you reach the 15-minute mark.

Like I mentioned earlier, adjust the intensity of the exercise and the run-walk ratios as needed to accommodate your current fitness level. Maybe you can only run at 7 mph for the first 3 rounds and then you have to go down to 6 mph— that's perfectly fine.

Work on improving on that every time you do the cardio workout. Next time you do the HIIT workout, try to go 4 rounds before you have to go down to 6 mph.

Or maybe you need to walk for longer than a minute in order to fully recuperate; if so, then do it! Remember that, just like with the weight training, the same principle of progressive overload still applies here.

We want to improve our cardiovascular fitness as time goes on.

How to Make HIIT Even More Effective (Yes It's Possible!)

Once you've done the HIIT for 15 minutes, there's something you can do right after that will help to make it even more effective—do 10-15 minutes of slow and steady state cardio immediately after the HIIT.

On its own, slow and steady state cardio isn't the best way to go about things as an endomorph. However, when you combine it with HIIT, something amazing happens.

When you do HIIT, you release free fatty acids into the bloodstream. Then the slow and steady state cardio will come in and burn off those free fatty acids.

If you just do the HIIT, then the free fatty acids will get reabsorbed. That's what makes this combo cardio workout of HIIT and steady state cardio so effective.

To do the steady state cardio, all you need to do is walk at the same pace for 10-15 minutes. For example, on a treadmill, you could walk at a pace of 3 mph for 10-15 minutes and that'll be enough to get the job done.

Here's a breakdown of the entire cardio workout done on a treadmill, which would take you around 25-30 minutes:

Part 1 HIIT:

High-Intensity Exercise for 30 seconds consisting of running on a treadmill at 7 mph.

Alternated with:

Low-Intensity Exercise for 1 minute consisting of walking on a treadmill at 3 mph.

Repeat for a total of 10 rounds until you reach the 15-minute mark.

Part 2 Steady State Cardio:

10-15 minutes of steady state cardio consisting of walking at 3 mph done immediately after the HIIT

Doing this cardio workout 2-3 times per week will be more than enough to start getting you some great results.

What if I Want to Lift Weights and Do Cardio?

Right now you might be wondering what you should do if you want to do both cardio and lift weights. The reality is that you can do cardio by itself or lift weights by itself.

You can do both cardio and lift weights, or you can even not exercise at all. Like I mentioned at the start of this chapter, it's possible to get results solely through your nutrition plan alone.

However, if you do want to lift weights and do cardio, then there's an optimal way to go about it. You have one of two choices—you can do your weight routine and cardio workout on the same day, or you can do them on separate days.

If you choose to do weights and cardio on the same day, then make sure that you do the weight routine first. The reason for this is because if you do cardio first, you may be fatigued, causing you to lift less weight than you normally would have if you were just starting a workout.

Lifting weights first won't cause too much of a performance decrease for your cardio workout. The other option you have is to do these workouts on separate days.

For example, on Mondays, Wednesdays, and Fridays you could lift weights. Then on Tuesdays, Thursdays, and Saturdays you could do cardio.

And if you only wanted to workout five days per week you could do that as well. You could still do the weight routine on Monday, Wednesday, and Friday.

And then you could do the cardio workout on Tuesdays and Thursdays. Do whatever works best for your schedule.

If you find it easy to go to the gym right after work for example, then exercising 5 days per week would be a good way to keep that schedule going. On the other hand, if you have a longer commute to get to the gym, then going less often but doing more when you're there is probably the better way to go.

What About Exercise in a Fasted State?

Fasting is a great and easy nutritional approach to help you burn fat. As it turns out, you can also use fasting to optimize the amount of fat that you burn in the gym.

If you've eaten a meal before working out, your body is in a fed state. This means that the main source of energy your body is going to use to fuel the workout is going to be glycogen.

Of course, if you're a performance athlete this will be beneficial. If you're an average individual who's looking to shed some weight, then we'll want to avoid this if possible.

When you workout in a fasted state, your body will be glycogen depleted. This doesn't mean that your body will totally shut down because it doesn't have any energy to use for the workout.

Instead, your body will have to go somewhere else in order to get the energy it needs to fuel the workout. And that somewhere else is going to be your fat stores.

By working out in a fasted state, you're essentially training your body to become more efficient at using fat for fuel instead of carbs.

Once you finish your workout, what should you do? Most people would say that you need to eat a post workout shake to help your body recover.

If you're an athlete concerned about performance, or someone whose priority is to build muscle, then yes, you should consume a post-workout meal. However, since the main goal is fat loss here, why do you feel obligated to eat something right after you worked out?

I think that the main reason for this is because supplement companies try to shove this idea down our throats. They act as if you have to consume post-workout protein or else your workout was a complete waste, and you're going to lose a lot of muscle.

This couldn't be further from the truth! When you exercise, your growth hormone levels will increase.

The growth hormone will help to save the muscle that you have, plus it'll help you burn more fat. However, when you consume a meal right after your workout, your growth hormone levels will be blunted and your insulin levels will increase.

This will cause you to stop burning fat so your body can instead start to process and store the calories you just ate.

That's why it's actually best if you delay eating anything if possible for 1-2 hours after you finish your workout.

This way you'll be able to take full advantage of the growth hormone increase. Not only that, but think about this logically—how does eating more calories help you lose more weight?

If this is an extra meal you're adding in simply for the sake of eating a post workout shake, how is that going to help you out? It won't!

Now I understand that working out in a fasted state and delaying a meal for 1-2 hours after you finish might not work for your schedule. The ideal way to be able to do this would be to workout early in the morning before you go to work.

If your first meal of the day is at 1:00 p.m. for example, then ideally you'd workout around 10:00 a.m. and finish around 11:00, and then have your meal at 1:00. However, if you can't workout until after you've eaten a meal, then don't sweat it.

Working out in a fasted state is the optimal way to do things for fat loss, but that doesn't mean you're better off not working out at all if you're going to be in a fed state. The same goes for delaying a meal for 1-2 hours after your workout is over.

For example, if you workout at noon and your first meal is usually at one, then go ahead and eat at that time. The main thing I advise against is going out of your way and eating an extra meal at a time when you usually wouldn't eat all because you feel like you have to.

If you finish your workout at a time when you would usually eat anyways, then go ahead and eat at that time.

Can I Add in Calories Burned Through Exercise to My Caloric Calculations?

You might also be wondering about the extra calories you'll be burning through exercise and if you can add those calories to your nutritional calculations. The answer to that is no, you can't.

The reason for this is because I want you to view the calories you burn through exercise as a bonus. These extra calories will either help you reach your goal that much faster or it'll help make up for any potential errors in your calculations.

Most people overestimate the number of calories they burn from exercise as well. This can totally mess up your nutritional calculations.

For example, you might think that you burned off 500 calories in the gym, when in reality you only burned off 250. You'll then eat an extra 250 calories when you shouldn't have, and that can hold you back from making progress.

Therefore, the best thing that you can do is to not factor in calories that you burn from exercise, and instead view them as a bonus.

Chapter 6: What You Need to Do to Ensure the Weight Stays Off

You might have the fear that, even if you are able to lose weight, you'll slowly start to gain it back. In this chapter, I'm going to share with you some tips and strategies you can use to help make sure that once you do lose the weight, it'll stay off for good.

What is Your Goal Bodyweight?

The first thing that you need to figure out is your goal bodyweight. In other words, how much would you ideally want to weigh in order to feel satisfied?

Depending on how far away you are from achieving your goal, you may not know the answer to this. That's completely fine. Most people don't know how much they'd ideally like to weigh.

If this is the case for you, then simply take your best guess as to what you think you'd like to weigh. For example, if someone weighed 230 pounds, he might guess that his goal bodyweight is 170 pounds.

He could then set goals and start to work towards that goal of weighing 170 pounds. As time goes on and he gets closer and closer to his goal, he might realize that his target is off by a bit.

For example, once he gets to 180 pounds he could see that his target bodyweight is better at 175 than 170. Or maybe he gets to 170 and realizes that he be satisfied at 160.

The point is to take your best guess and then adjust as necessary. The only true way to know your goal bodyweight is to look at yourself in the mirror and see if you're happy with how you look.

If you are, then step on the scale and see how much you weigh. That's your goal bodyweight.

Obviously, you don't have a crystal ball to see what that number is, so take your best guess with where you're at right now. You can always adjust it later as you start making progress.

What Should You Do When You Reach Your Target Bodyweight?

When you do reach your goal bodyweight, how do things change? Should you keep doing things exactly as you were to lose weight in the first place?

Or should you go back to your old eating habits? As you can probably guess, you shouldn't go back to your old eating patterns.

Doing so will cause you to gain back the weight that you worked so hard to lose in the first place. Instead, you should continue eating in the same way that you did to lose the weight in the first place.

However, you won't be eating the same amount of calories. Let's say for example you were eating 2,200 calories per day in order to lose 1 pound per week.

Now that you've reached your goal bodyweight, you no longer need to continue eating in a caloric deficit. You're now going to eat at your maintenance caloric intake.

This is because you now want to maintain your new bodyweight instead of continuing to lose weight. To figure out what your current maintenance calories are, simply find out how large of a deficit your were creating and add that number back to your current caloric intake.

For example, if you were eating 2,200 calories a day in order to lose 1 pound per week, this would mean that you were eating at a deficit of 500 calories per day. You would simply take 2,200 and add 500 to that number to reach 2,700 calories per day.

This is how many calories you'll need to eat every day to maintain your new bodyweight. This is pretty cool!

You now get to enjoy eating some more calories without having to worry about the weight coming back. You still want to be mindful of how much you're eating though.

It can be easy to get carried away and overeat. That's why you want to make sure that you're still measuring your calories and macros.

With that being said, what's the best way to go about adding in those additional calories? It's not wise to add an additional meal to your diet plan.

For example, if you're currently eating 3 meals per day, then stick with that. Don't bump that up to 4 meals per day.

The reason for this is because those extra calories might not be enough to justify eating another meal. This might cause you to overeat, and we want to avoid that at all costs.

Instead, a better idea is to add more to the meals that you're currently eating. For example, you could eat an additional side dish for one of your meals.

Or you could eat 250 calories more of a side dish for two of your meals. You can break it up however you like as long as you're accurately accounting for everything that you eat.

And like I mentioned earlier, your eating patterns need to stay the same. This means that if you were fasting for 16 hours a day, eating a moderate amount of carbs, and eating healthy foods 85% of the time, then you need to continue doing those things.

If you start to deviate from what made you successful in the first place, then you'll start gaining the weight back. This is why sustainability is key.

If it's too hard to follow a diet plan, you won't be able to maintain your goal bodyweight. This endomorph nutrition plan is set up in a way to make it easy for you to continue the plan once you're satisfied with where you're at.

At the end of the day, you need to remember that you must make some sort of sacrifice in order to get results and keep them. You can't be sedentary, eat what you want, when you want to, in any amount that you want and expect to be happy with your fitness results.

A sacrifice has to be made somewhere. The more willing you are to make sacrifices, the better off you'll be. You don't need to go crazy, but there has to be some give somewhere.

With this diet plan, we're sacrificing when you can eat, and the overall amount that you can eat for the day. This is the easiest thing to surrender.

You don't have to completely give up certain foods, and you don't have to exercise if you don't want to. Do take note that, even though this nutrition plan is made to be as easy as possible, it still requires you to give up some things in order to get you to where you want to go.

Make no mistake about it, getting in shape requires discipline and effort for a prolonged period of time.

Chapter 7: Endomorph Supplement Guide

In this chapter, I'm going to share with you everything you need to know about supplements. Supplements are a very popular topic among fitness enthusiasts, but it's also a confusing one.

By the end of this chapter, you'll know exactly what supplements can help you out along the way and which ones you should avoid. Let's get started...

The Correct Way to Think About Supplements

The supplement industry is a multibillion-dollar industry. That sure is a lot of money, and sadly, a lot of supplement companies may not have your best interest at heart.

They might try to sell you on something that isn't backed by very much research and is mostly hype. And if you aren't properly educated on supplements, it can be very easy to fall for the hype.

This is why it's so critical that you think of supplements in the correct way. What is a supplement anyway?

It's meant to be a tool that enhances something when the supplement is added to it. For example, a supplement is meant to enhance a proper exercise and nutrition plan.

However, most people don't view supplements in this manner. Instead, they view supplements as something that is meant to replace a proper diet and exercise routine.

As if the supplement can do all of the work for them. And this isn't uncommon.

Most people who buy weight loss supplements aren't doing it to supplement a proper nutrition plan. Instead, they're hoping to lose weight without having to put forth any effort, similar to a get rich quick scheme.

Like I said, billions of dollars are being made here and yet the obesity epidemic is only getting worse. It can be so easy to fall for the magical hype of a new weight loss supplement.

You'll see a commercial for a new weight loss pill, and you'll see all of these people who supposedly lost weight using it. So you buy into it, all while ignoring the little asterisk on the bottom of the screen that says something like "participants used this pill alongside a proper diet and exercise plan."

That's why the first lesson you need to understand when it comes to supplements is that there is nothing magical about them. They're meant to add to a proper diet and exercise plan, not replace them.

At the end of the day, it's still going to require dedicated effort and persistence in order to reach your goals. There is no getting around that. Supplement companies know that you have to work hard to reach your goals, but they prey on people who want to take a shortcut.

People will wonder what the harm is in trying the product; it's only $20. If it doesn't work, then I lose $20, but if it does work, then I'll get in shape without having to put forth any effort.

The reward greatly outweighs the risk. This is a similar mentality people have when playing the lottery.

Even though the odds of you winning are extremely slim, millions of people still play the lottery every year for the hope that they can get rich without having to work for it. The risk of wasting $2 on a lottery ticket is well worth the potential reward of winning millions, even if that chance is quite slim.

The second thing you need to understand about supplements is that no supplement is required in order for you to reach your fitness goal. If someone says that supplement x is a must-have in order to lose weight, then they're not telling the truth.

The truth is that you don't need any supplements in order to get in better shape. I want you to be able to experience this truth first hand.

That's why for the first 6 weeks that you're doing the diet program, you're not allowed to take any supplements. I want you to see that it is possible to get results without having to take any supplements.

Then once that 6-week period is up, you can take some of the supplements that I'll recommend later in the chapter. This is a great way to go about doing things because you'll get into the habit of following the nutrition plan before taking any supplements.

Most people do the exact opposite of this. They decide that they want to start a new fitness routine.

Then they immediately go to the supplement store and buy a bunch of supplements before they've actually even started their plan! Then time goes by and they never get around to starting their nutrition plan and the supplements sit there and collect dust.

Doing things the other way around proves to yourself that you're dedicated enough to actually get some benefits out of supplements if you use them. This should come as a relief.

You don't have to worry about spending extra money on supplements if you don't want to, or if you don't have room in your budget for them. Usually, it's the simplest things that work best, such as eating right and exercising.

However, that doesn't necessarily mean simple is easy. The third tip when it comes to supplements is to buy what you can afford in terms of importance.

While you may not want to completely skip out on supplements, you might only be able to afford one supplement. That's completely fine.

Don't feel as if you have to buy multiple supplements in order for them to be worth it. I'll be sharing with you the benefits of different popular supplements and which ones to get first if you're on a limited budget.

Finally, if everything else is in order, what kind of a difference can you expect supplements to make? I'd say that the right supplements, when paired in conjunction with a good diet plan, could make around a 5-10% difference at most.

So you can look at that however you like. You certainly can't get around the fact that 90-95% of your results are coming from your nutrition and exercise plan.

However, if you want that last little boost, supplements could be the thing to help you get there. With that being said, let's get into what supplements are worth your money and which ones aren't...

Supplements You Should Avoid

Here are some popular supplements that you should avoid at all costs, even though they're quite popular. Don't buy into the hype with these supplements because they're just that—hype!

Testosterone boosters

Testosterone is a male sex hormone that is responsible for sex drive, strength, muscle size, bone mass, and distribution of fat. This isn't to say that only men have testosterone; women have testosterone too.

However, women have much less testosterone than men do. With all of these benefits, it's easy to see why testosterone boosters are a very popular supplement for men.

The way this supplement is presented makes people think that they can get similar benefits to steroids without any negative consequences. The truth is that this supplement is a bunch of hype and not much more.

Most testosterone boosters will use one or more of the following ingredients—ZMA, D-aspartic acid, and tribulus terrestris. The research shows that at best D-aspartic acid can temporarily increase testosterone levels (4).

Multiple studies show that tribulus terrestris doesn't have any effect on testosterone levels (5). What tribulus terrestris will do is increase libido, which will make you think that the supplement is really working.

ZMA is only effective at increasing testosterone levels if you're deficient in zinc to begin with (6). Testosterone boosters aren't a good route to go if you want to increase your testosterone levels.

However, there are a few things you can do if you want to naturally increase your testosterone levels. The first is to improve your body composition.

There's a correlation between body composition levels and testosterone. Correlation doesn't mean causation. However, as you start to lean down, this should mean your testosterone levels will start to go up some.

The other thing that you can do is regularly lift weights, as this has been shown to help increase testosterone levels as well (7). You're going to be following a sound nutrition plan and exercise plan if you choose to exercise.

Therefore, you really have nothing to worry about in regards to your testosterone levels. Just focus on the main task at hand, which is reaching your goal bodyweight, and you'll be good to go.

Fat Burners

Most fat burner supplements are a waste of your money. It's a little ironic that a supplement specifically designed to help you lose weight fails miserably at what it's supposed to do.

They'll use a variety of different ingredients that are allegedly going to help you boost your metabolism and suppress your appetite, among other claims. Here are some of the ingredients you may find in fat burners, and why they're not effective at what they claim to do:

Hoodia

This comes from a desert cactus in countries in Africa. It's supposed to help blunt your appetite, therefore allowing you to lose weight because you wouldn't be eating as much.

However, hoodia is not only ineffective at suppressing your appetite, it can also be harmful to your body by causing an increase in blood pressure (8).

Vitamin B12

This is a vitamin that helps to convert foods we eat into energy and it helps with the formation of red blood cells. Some claim that B12 can help to increase weight loss because of the boost in energy that it can provide.

However, this may only be the case for individuals who have a deficiency in vitamin B12 to begin with. There's not sufficient evidence to show that taking more B12 is beneficial to weight loss for individuals who already have normal B12 levels (9).

Garcinia Cambogia

This ingredient comes from the tropical fruit tamarind. It's supposed to help limit the production of fat in the body and suppress appetite.

However, there's not conclusive evidence to help support that these claims are anything more than temporary at best (10).

BCAA's

If you're going to be working out in a fasted state, then you may feel the need to buy BCAA's. The main selling point behind them is that they can help prevent excessive muscle breakdown during your workouts.

I almost fell for the hype on this supplement back in college, but fortunately they were too expensive, and I couldn't afford to waste my money on them! BCAA's stand for branch chained amino acids, and they're essentially the broken down form of protein.

This allows them to be more easily digested and utilized by the body faster than protein. Eating food before you train spikes your insulin; however, amino acids have a much smaller impact on your insulin levels.

Therefore, you can take amino acids before your workout and still train in a fasted state. The amino acid leucine is the most effective one at preventing muscle breakdown.

However, you have to think about the cost here. Is it really worth investing in amino acids (which can be quite expensive) to ensure you're not losing muscle?

Remember, if you're already eating an adequate amount of protein every day and you're not super lean to begin with, then your body will want to use fat for fuel instead of protein (i.e. your muscle).

If you're already very lean and not getting in a lot of protein, then BCAA's probably would be worth it if you're exercising in a fasted state. For most people though, it's not going to be worth the money.

Pre Workout Supplements

This is another supplement that's extremely popular nowadays. The idea behind this supplement is that it'll help to increase the intensity of your workouts, allowing you to burn more calories and lose more weight.

Yes, most pre-workout supplements do contain some beneficial ingredients such as citrulline malate, but again is it worth the cost, especially considering what your goals are? The reason why I say this is because you could be paying for ingredients that help you increase muscle size and strength, like creatine.

Creatine is a great supplement, but if your main goal is fat loss, do you really want to pay for something that won't help you reach your primary goal? Additionally, pre-workout supplements commonly contain arginine AKG (AAKG) which helps to provide better blood flow to the muscles.

In the fitness world, this is referred to as getting a pump. You don't have to get a pump to gain strength or build muscle, and you certainly don't need to get a pump to burn fat.

It may look and feel good, but its tangible benefits are questionable. Not only that, but do you want to become reliant on something in order to have a good workout?

Imagine that you're about to go to the gym, but then you realize you're out of your pre-workout supplement, so you decide to workout later after you can go to the store. Chances are good that you'll never get around to completing that workout.

You're now relying on your pre-workout supplement as a crutch, and it'll start dictating how good your workouts are, or if they will even happen in the first place. Even with this being the case, you still might be interested in taking something like a pre-workout.

There's a much cheaper option that I'll be sharing with you in the recommended supplements section. This will provide you with many of the same benefits that the expensive pre-workout supplements will at only a fraction of the cost.

Multivitamins

Maybe you're like me and you grew up taking a multivitamin with breakfast. My chewable multivitamin tasted good, and my mom told me it would help me stay healthy so I actually enjoyed taking it.

Now though, there are much better things I'd rather spend my money on. A multivitamin contains of a bunch of different micronutrients.

These are things our bodies need in small amounts in order to survive. Conversely, macronutrients like protein, carbs, and fat are things our bodies need in large amounts in order to properly function.

This is what makes multivitamins seem like they're such a great supplement. All you have to do is take a pill and it'll help make up for any vitamin deficiencies that you may have.

This begs the question of whether or not most people are deficient with a lot of the vitamins contained in these multivitamin pills? Are we once again being sold something that we don't really need?

Some multivitamins will claim that they can help prevent certain diseases or illnesses like cardiovascular disease. However, you have to consider how healthy the individual is to begin with.

Someone who's already eating a healthy diet and exercising regularly isn't going to need a multivitamin to help prevent certain diseases. On the other hand, someone who's nutrient deficient would need to take in more of certain vitamins and minerals.

Then again, is a multivitamin the best way to go about doing this? It would be better if the person instead focused on improving his or her diet by eating more wholesome foods.

Not only would this save you money, but consuming vitamins and minerals from whole food sources is better absorbed by the body than consuming them via a pill. Most individuals in counties where there is an overabundance of food are probably not deficient in most of the vitamins that are contained in a multivitamin pill.

Therefore, multivitamins aren't worth it for most people. The body will simply secrete most of the excess not needed through urine.

Not only that but taking a multivitamin might make you feel as if it's okay for you to eat more junk food than you should because the multivitamin will help make up for it. If you follow the nutrition principles as they're laid out in this book, then you shouldn't have any need for a multivitamin.

Sadly, the multivitamin supplement is something a lot of people fall for because it makes us feel better about ourselves. It makes us feel like we're taking a proactive step in taking care of our health.

And depending on how deficient you are, then maybe you actually could be. Chances are good though that the multivitamin pill isn't benefiting you much, and your money would be better spent elsewhere.

Digestive Enzymes

This is a supplement that I've recommended in the past, however upon further study I've realized that this supplement is meant more for specific individuals with digestive problems, such as irritable bowel syndrome.

Taking digestive enzymes won't be worth it for most people. Enzymes are found in certain foods (such as fruits and vegetables) and they're produced by the body.

Whenever we eat food, enzymes will help to break down the food so that the body can absorb it. For example, protein will get broken down into amino acids, carbs will get broken down into glucose, and fat will get broken down into fatty acids.

Our bodies have specific enzymes that help to break down each of these macronutrients and many others. The idea behind taking the supplement is that it can help you absorb more of the nutrients from the foods that you're eating.

This is important because what you eat technically isn't as important as what you absorb. Remember that your body releases the enzymes necessary to break down the foods that you're eating.

If you're getting your enzymes from an outside supplement, then over time your body will stop naturally producing enzymes because it no longer needs to. This is similar to when a male takes steroids to boost testosterone.

Over time the testes will stop naturally producing testosterone because the body is getting sufficient amounts from an outside source. If you're not currently suffering from any digestive issues, then the best thing you can do to maximize enzyme production and help improve your digestive health is to slow down and chew your food properly.

Most people only chew their food 3-4 times before swallowing. This is a problem because as you chew, your body releases enzymes to help your body digest that food.

If you don't spend enough time properly chewing your food, then you're not giving your body much of a chance to release the necessary enzymes to break down that food. Instead, you want to chew slowly and enough times to where the food is almost liquidly before you swallow.

This means you'll chew your food around 30 times before swallowing. Not only will this help improve your digestion, but it can also help you lose more weight by consuming less food.

When you eat faster, you might wind up consuming more calories because it can take 20 minutes from the time you start eating for the stomach to signal to the brain that you're full and to stop eating. Therefore, most people are better off slowing down and properly chewing their food rather than taking a digestive enzyme.

Detox Supplements

This is a supplement that's been gaining a lot of popularity in recent years. The selling point is that your body contains a lot of toxins that need to be dispelled of.

By using a special detox kit, you can help to cleanse your body of harmful toxins that are holding you back from losing weight. The problem is that different detox supplements are made by different companies, and these companies can't seem to agree on exactly what a toxin is.

This makes it hard to know what the supplement is trying to get rid of and how it's getting rid of it. Some detox supplements contain a polymerizing agent that causes your poop to stick together.

This can cause you to excrete one large piece of stool when you use the bathroom. This may lead you to think the supplement is really making a difference, when it reality it isn't doing anything to truly help you.

This might be the reason why some people claim that they feel better after going on a detox. The truth is that it could very well be a placebo instead of something the supplement actually did.

Your body is already set up with organs like the liver and kidneys that are designed to help filter and get rid of waste in the body. This isn't to say you should go wild and overload these organs by eating junk food all of the time, or excessively drink and smoke.

Instead, you can help support these organs in your body by living a proper healthy lifestyle. You can do this by making sure that you're eating lots of wholesome foods, getting plenty of sleep, and exercising.

Supplements That Are Worth Your Money

Now it's time to get into what you should be buying if you want to invest some money into supplements. They're going to be listed in order of importance; however, certain supplements may suit your individual needs better.

At the end of the day, I recommend going with what will best fit your budget and your needs.

Protein Powder

The first supplement that I would recommend getting is protein powder. The reason for it is rather simple—convenience.

Having protein powder makes it so much easier to reach your daily protein intake. Not only that, but if you find yourself in a pinch without any healthy foods to eat, protein powder can be an easy way to consume quality calories.

Make no mistake about it, there's nothing special about the protein that's in protein powder. It's simply protein in a powder form.

This is true regardless of what various supplement companies will tell you. The main thing you want to focus on is making sure you're getting an adequate amount of protein.

Sometimes it can be hard to reach your daily protein macros solely from whole food sources. Ideally, you'd get all the protein you need from whole foods.

When you can't though, this is where protein powder really shines. You can easily make a protein shake or mix the powder in with some other food like cottage cheese or plain greek yogurt.

This can be part of a healthy high protein meal. Compare this to eating protein from whole foods, such as lean meats like chicken or beef.

You have to buy the meat, then prepare it, cook it, eat it, and clean up afterwards. If you find yourself in a pinch for time, or maybe you're away from your house, then protein powder will come in handy.

The thing you want to watch out for is something known as protein guilt. This is where you consume more protein than necessary for fear of losing muscle, or because you think that you have to eat a certain amount of protein with every meal.

Remember that the goal is to lose weight. Consuming more calories than necessary (even if they're from protein) will take you farther away from your goal, not closer to it.

Of course, 40% of your total calories will be coming from protein, so it's unlikely that you'll overeat it. Regardless, it's still something you want to be aware of.

Not all protein powder is created equally though. You'll definitely want to make sure that you get the correct protein powder to help suit your needs.

The first thing you need to find out is what type of protein powder you'll want to get. Whey protein is the most common type of protein on the market.

It's a milk-based type of protein and it tends to be the cheapest type of protein you can buy. There are many other different kinds of protein powder such as soy, beef, hemp, egg, and pea protein, among others.

Unless you have some type of allergy to dairy or you're lactose intolerant, then sticking with whey protein is going to be your best bet. If you do have an allergy or are lactose intolerant, then going with something like an egg protein would probably be your best option.

Yes, this is going to be more expensive than something like a whey protein, but it's a very high-quality type of protein that you'll be able to consume without issues. As far as whey protein is concerned, there are three main kinds that you can get—concentrate, isolate, and hydrolysate.

Whey concentrate is the cheapest of the three kinds. This is because whey concentrate contains a lower percentage of protein than the other two kinds.

A good concentrate will contain around 70-80% of the total calories per serving from protein. The rest will be made up of carbs and fat. This is the type of protein that I've used for years, and it's worked great for me.

The other two types of whey protein may suit your needs better though. The next type of whey protein is whey isolate.

Whey isolate contains a higher percentage of protein and fewer carbs and fat. Typically, whey isolate contains around 90% of the total calories per serving from protein, which is pretty good.

If you're willing to pay a bit more money, this could be a better option for you, especially if you want to avoid the extra carbs and fat the concentrate contains.

Finally, we have whey hydrolysate. This is the most expensive of the three kinds of whey protein. It's a predigested protein which means that it'll get absorbed by the body the fastest.

This may be something to consider if your primary goal is to build muscle; however, it won't serve much of a use for fat loss purposes, especially for how much more expensive it is.

When you're looking to buy a protein powder, there are some things that you're going to want to watch out for. This will mostly apply for when you're looking to buy a whey concentrate protein powder.

Be that as it may, it still doesn't hurt to double check these things when buying an isolate or hydrolysate protein. The first thing you want to check is the ingredient list.

The first ingredient on the label should be protein or protein blend. That may seem obvious, but that isn't always the case with some protein powders.

Some protein powders are made with cheap fillers such as maltodextrin. If something like maltodextrin is the first ingredient on the label, then you should avoid buying that protein powder.

The next thing you want to be on the lookout for is something known as a proprietary blend. You may notice the words proprietary blend on the nutrition info on the protein powder.

The specific amount of any ingredient listed under the proprietary blend doesn't have to be listed. For someone who knows what to look for, this definitely makes it seem like the company is trying to hide something.

The proprietary blend could list mostly high-quality ingredients and one cheap filler ingredient. Since the amount isn't listed, the blend could consist mostly of that one cheap ingredient and you'd have no way of knowing.

And since most people don't know what a proprietary blend is, this will even get marketed as a good thing sometimes. Some companies will try to use the proprietary blend to help increase the perceived value of their product.

When you see the words 'proprietary blend' on a protein powder label, you should not buy that protein. There's simply no way to tell if something is trying to be covered up.

A reputable company won't try to hide any of their ingredients or the amounts of those ingredients that are contained in their protein powder. The next thing you'll want to check for is the percentage of protein the powder contains.

If you're buying a whey protein concentrate, then you want to make sure the protein contains no less than 70% of the total calories per serving from protein. Ideally, this number would be 80%, but as long as it's 70% and above, you'll be okay.

Anything lower than 70% means that you're not getting your money's worth. You're likely paying for cheap filler carbs that aren't going to help you reach your goal.

To figure this out, look at the nutritional info and see how many calories per serving the powder contains. Then look at the serving size for the protein, which is typically going to be in grams.

Take that number and multiply it by four to convert it into calories. Then divide the protein calories by the total calories to get your percentage. For example:

220 total calories per serving

40 grams of protein per serving

40x4=160

160/220= .73 which converts to 73%

This means that this protein powder contains 73% of the total calories from protein, so it passes the test. The last thing that you want to look out for is something known as amino acid spiking.

This is where companies will spike their formulas with cheap amino acids in order to get a higher protein reading during testing. This allows them to get away with putting higher amounts of protein on the label than the powder actually contains.

Of course, companies aren't going to blatantly put on their label that they spike their formula. Therefore, it's up to you to do your own research and make sure that you're buying from a trustworthy company.

Ultimately, if a protein powder passes all of these four tests, then it's a good protein powder and worth buying. Yes, there is quite a bit to look out for when it comes to buying protein, but doing your homework will pay off.

Protein powder is one of the most popular supplements out there. That kind of status attracts companies who will do shady things in order to get your money.

Fish Oil

The next supplement on the recommended list is going to be fish oil. There are two different kinds of essential fatty acids—Omega 6 and Omega 3 fatty acids.

Our bodies don't make these fatty acids, so we must consume them through our diets. Omega 6 fatty acids are an inflammatory fatty acid.

This aspect of Omega 6's isn't bad in and of itself. In fact, it's important for a properly functioning immune system.

The problem occurs when things get out of balance and we consume too many Omega 6's in comparison to Omega 3's. Foods that are commonly high in Omega 6 fatty acids include various types of nuts such as walnuts and different oils like soybean oil.

Omega 3 fatty acids, on the other hand, act as an anti-inflammatory in the body. These are found commonly in foods such as fish, chia seeds, and flax seeds.

Anti-inflammatories are important for preventing chronic diseases. In fact, any disease that ends in the suffix -itis is caused by an excessive amount of inflammation in a certain area. For example, arthritis is an inflammation of the joints.

Omega 3 fatty acids can help improve heart health; research has shown that Omega 3 fatty acids can increase HDL cholesterol, which is the good kind of cholesterol.

Some studies also show that supplementing with Omega 3's can help boost your metabolism (11). However, this is a slight boost at best, and it's definitely nothing that will be able to replace a proper diet and exercise routine.

The main reason to supplement with fish oil isn't for any potential weight loss benefits. It's more so for your overall health.

Most Americans consume way more Omega 6 fatty acids than Omega 3 fatty acids; this is where problems can arise. By supplementing with Omega 3 fatty acids, you'll help close that gap and keep your body from becoming chronically inflamed.

This will allow you to stay healthy and be able to focus your attention on your weight loss goals. It's hard to do that if you're feeling sick.

As with most supplements, quality is going to be key here. A lot of the fish oils on the market are low grade and aren't going to be worth your money.

So what should you look out for when buying this supplement? The first thing is going to be how the oil is being extracted from the fish during the manufacturing process.

You want to make sure the supplement uses cold pressed manufacturing techniques in order to extract the oil. Cheaper fish oils that use heat to extract the oil from the fish can lead to oxidative damage.

This can cause more inflammation to arise in your body, which defeats the purpose of taking the supplement in the first place. The next thing you want to make sure of is that the fish used were caught from the wild and not from farm-raised fish.

Wild fish will be of a better quality than farm-raised fish. Thirdly, you want to check to make sure that the fish oil supplement is certified for purity by a third party.

You don't want the fish oil to contain an excessive amount of toxins. Ideally, a fish oil supplement should contain no more than 100 parts per billion mercury, 100 parts per billion PCB's, 100 parts per billion arsenic, and 2 parts per trillion dioxins and furans.

Finally, you want to check how much EPA and DHA are contained in the supplement. EPA and DHA are the main Omega 3 fatty acids that you're after.

Some fish oil supplements will be sneaky and say that their supplement contains 1,000 mg of fish oil per serving. Yet the total EPA and DHA might only be 250 mg of that 1,000 mg.

Essentially, the total amount of fish oil per serving doesn't matter. You should instead focus on how much EPA and DHA the supplement contains. That's why you must carefully read the label before buying.

Ideally, you want to aim for around 1,800 to 3,000 mg of EPA and DHA per day depending on your needs. This is a total amount between the two, not a recommendation for each one.

For example, if you were taking 1,800 mg daily, you might consume 900 mg of EPA's and 900 mg of DHA's. Of course, this doesn't all have to come from supplementation.

You can get some or all of your Omega 3's from your diet. It's similar to the protein powder.

If you find it hard to get an adequate amount of Omega 3's in your diet, then consider supplementing with them for the sake of convenience.

You may also be wondering about krill oil; it is quite similar to fish oil in the sense that it's an Omega 3 supplement that contains EPA's and DHA's. However, there are a few differences between the two.

For starters, krill oil contains the antioxidant known as astaxanthin, which is rarely found in fish oil. Antioxidants are important for combating free radicals, improving skin health, and supporting a healthy immune system, among other things.

These are some great benefits; however, that's about the only major benefit you'll get from taking krill oil over fish oil. Thanks to the marketing around astaxanthin, krill oil tends to be more expensive per serving than fish oil does.

Not only that, but many krill oils actually contain less EPA's and DHA's per serving than fish oils do! This isn't always the case, but always make sure you check the labels before you buy.

If you have to spend more money to get an adequate amount of EPA's and DHA's, then it's not worth it. You're taking the supplement for the EPA's and the DHA's, not to get the antioxidant astaxanthin.

If you want to get more antioxidants in your body, then eat more foods such as blueberries, strawberries, walnuts, and kale.

Caffeine

The last recommended supplement on the list is also the cheapest—caffeine. Caffeine can help to give you a boost in energy by blocking a neurotransmitter known as adenosine.

This boost in energy can help increase exercise intensity, allowing you to burn more calories at the gym. This is the better pre-workout supplement that I alluded to earlier and the reason why is simple.

Caffeine gives you very similar benefits to that of a pre-workout, yet it's only a fraction of the cost per serving. You can drink coffee or even take it in the form of a caffeine pill before your workout to help increase performance.

There is also some research out there to show that caffeine can help to boost your metabolism (12). However, don't expect anything too crazy from this.

Remember that supplements only make a small difference when paired in conjunction with a proper diet and exercise plan. Everyone would be in great shape if all you had to do was drink coffee before heading off to work.

Finally, if you're already a coffee drinker, I want to advise that you to stick as closely to pure black coffee as you can. The more sugar, creamer, and milk you add to the coffee, the worse off the beverage is going to be for you.

Any boost in metabolism the coffee does provide to you will quickly be erased by the extra calories you're consuming, thus defeating the purpose.

You probably noticed that the list of recommended supplements was much shorter than the list you should avoid. That wasn't by accident; most supplements on the market aren't that good.

And the ones that I do recommend aren't going to be able to do all of the work for you. Don't ever get mistaken by the fact that most of the time supplements sell because of hype and the hope that they might work.

It can be easy to fall for the latest craze of a new supplement that just hit the market. However, the vast majority of new supplements that come out aren't going to be worth it.

So if you're interested in checking out a new supplement, use the test of time. See how the long the supplement has been around for.

For example, protein powder has been around for a while, and it's not going anywhere anytime soon. On the other hand, if a brand new fat burner came out last week, hold off on buying it.

See if it'll still be around 3-5 years later and if there is science is to back it up. The test of time doesn't guarantee a supplement to be worth it, but it's a good place to start.

At the end of the day, make sure that you always do a thorough amount of research on the supplement and the brand before you buy.

Chapter 8: Frequently Asked Questions

What Can I Drink While I'm Fasting?

When you're fasting, you should only drink beverages that contain zero calories. Most of the time, this means that you're going to be drinking water, which is how it should be.

You can always use a water enhancer to add a little flavor to the water if you prefer that. Aside from water, black coffee and green tea are also an option for you to drink during your fasting periods.

The main thing is that the drink does not contain any calories. If it does, that drink can break your fast, and we don't want that to happen.

Drinking diet sodas would therefore be acceptable, however, I recommend avoiding them if possible. Diet soda contains artificial sweeteners like aspartame and saccharin in them.

There's also research to show that diet soda may spark dopamine in the brain and fuel hormones that cause hunger (13). This can lead to an increase in appetite.

That's something you'll definitely want to avoid when you're trying to fast for a certain length of time. You may drink diet soda and not notice any difference in your appetite. Even if this is the case, it is clear that diet soda does not provide your diet any nutritional value.

That's why you should stick with water as much as possible, even if the taste is bland. If you're currently drinking a lot of soda right now, do your best to slowly wean yourself off of it.

Don't try to quit cold turkey. If you try to do that, it'll make things feel overwhelming, and most likely cause you to start drinking them again.

For example, if you're drinking 20 ounces of soda per day, start by trying to scale that back to 16 ounces per day. Then a week later, go down to 12 ounces; continue this pattern until you get to zero.

Drinking 20 ounces of soda per day is around 240 calories and 65 grams of sugar! And since those are empty calories, they aren't going to do anything to help keep you full.

They're simply going to take away from other foods that you could be eating. That's why it's really important to get to the point where you're drinking water the majority of the time.

How Many Meals Should I Eat Per Day?

There's a myth that eating 6 small meals throughout the day will help to boost your metabolism. Research shows that meal frequency does not affect weight loss (14).

This means that it doesn't matter whether you eat 6 meals, 3 meals, or just one meal a day; your weight loss will not be affected as long as you're still eating the same overall amount of calories.

This means that you can eat however many meals a day that works best for you and your schedule. Since you're going to be doing the fasting protocol, this means you're probably going to be eating 2 or 3 meals per day.

Doing anything more than that will be hard to squeeze into an eight-hour feeding window. In addition to that, the meals would likely be so small that they might not fill you up very well.

Eating fewer meals will allow you to eat larger and more satisfying meals. It's up to you if you'd rather eat two or three meals a day.

In an earlier chapter, I gave the example of fasting until noon and then eating three meals—one at noon, one at 4:00, and one at 8:00. If you prefer, you could eat only two meals during that eight-hour feeding window instead of three.

For example, you could eat at noon and 6:00 p.m, or maybe 1:00 p.m. and 7:00 p.m.

You can break it up however you like. When you eat, you might enjoy feasting on larger meals, in which case 2 meals per day would be more up your alley.

Or maybe you're able to better control how much you eat if you consume 3 meals a day. Again, simply do whatever works best for you and your schedule.

How Should You Divide Up Calories Across Your Meals?

Let's say you're eating 2,100 calories per day across 3 meals in order to lose weight. You might think that you need to eat 700 calories per meal, but you certainly don't have to do things that way if you don't want to.

You can divide up your calories across your meals in whatever way that you like. For example, if you usually don't like eating that big of a lunch, you could eat a smaller lunch and save some of those extra calories for later in the day during dinner.

Your first meal could contain 400 calories, your second meal 1,000, and your final meal 700. This still works out to the same 2,100 calorie total for the day.

The point is to break things up in a way that works best for you and your schedule. Remember, we're focused on the long haul here.

If it's easier for you to eat more calories during one meal and less during another, then definitely do that!

What Should I Do If I Find It Hard to Adapt to Fasting When I First Start?

When most people first start fasting, they find it to be rather difficult. This should come as no surprise because most of us have been eating breakfast our whole lives.

Our bodies have been trained to expect a meal in the morning soon after we wake up. However, if our bodies can be trained to expect a meal soon after waking, then that means we can also train our bodies to expect the first meal to come later in the day.

While this initial transition period may not be fun, think of what will happen when you make it to the other side. You'll be used to delaying your first meal of the day, and you'll be able to fast with ease.

In fact, it really won't feel like a diet at that point. It would be harder to quit and go back to eating breakfast than it would be to continue skipping it.

With that being said though, how do you reach that point? Well, the first thing you need to understand is that it can take about 2-4 weeks in order for you to fully adapt to your new fasting protocol.

This is definitely something you'll want to keep in mind. Initially, when you're first starting out, you might want to quit because it seems like this will never end.

However, it will end. The hunger you're feeling will only be temporary.

Once you make it to the other side, those feelings of hunger in the morning will stop persisting. Therefore, always keep in mind that you can do this for 2-4 weeks, and you'll be good to go for a very long time to come. It won't last forever.

Aside from that mental tip, the first thing you want to make sure you're doing is drinking enough water upon waking up. The reason for this is because you haven't had any water during the night while you were sleeping.

This means that you're going to be dehydrated when you wake up. Sometimes our bodies will confuse our dehydration with hunger.

This is known as false hunger. There's a chance that you could be eating breakfast when you're not even actually hungry—you could simply be dehydrated!

That's why it's critical that you drink a couple of glasses of water as soon as you can after waking up. Even after that, make sure you're drinking plenty of water throughout the day.

The best way to be able to tell if you're dehydrated or not is to go by the color of your urine. If your urine is more of a yellow color, then that means you're dehydrated.

If it's clear, you're hydrated. This is the first step you need to take in order to make adapting to fasting easier.

Sadly, even though everyone wakes up dehydrated, most people still don't drink nearly enough water in the morning or throughout the day! After that, the next thing you may want to consider doing is drinking black coffee.

Coffee can help to blunt your appetite, and it can also help to give you a small boost in metabolism as I mentioned earlier. Even if you're not a regular coffee drinker, this may be something you'll want to try if you notice that it makes the adjustment phase easier.

Finally, the last thing you can do if you notice that you're hungry before it's time to eat is to chew gum. Make sure that the gum is sugar-free, and that it contains 5 or fewer calories.

We don't want to consume anything that could break our fast earlier than wanted, which includes chewing gum. You might not think that chewing gum would do much, but it surprisingly does.

The first reason why it helps so much is because it distracts you. You're not focusing as much on your hunger as you are on chewing the gum.

Not only that, but you can't eat anything if you have a piece of gum in your mouth. Yes, you could simply spit the gum out and eat something, but for some weird reason you might find that you won't want to eat anything until you're done chewing the piece of gum.

Psychologically, this could be because of something that is known as a sunk cost. You spent money on the gum, and you want to get the maximum value out of it.

You don't want to feel as if you wasted your money on gum that you barely chewed. If you spat it out after 5 minutes to eat something, then it wouldn't feel like you got much value out of it.

That's why chewing gum can be so powerful. You just have to get started with it, and it could be 30 minutes before you're ready to spit it out.

And by that point, you may have forgotten that you're even hungry! Finally, once you're done chewing the gum, you're going to have a minty fresh breath that you may not be so eager to ruin by eating something.

Yes, chewing gum may be a sneaky little tactic, but do whatever tricks work in the beginning to get the job done.

The last thing you want to make sure you're doing is keeping yourself busy. Distract yourself however you can.

The more bored you are, the more your mind is going to remind you of how hungry you are. Think of a time in the past, a time when you did something so fun that you forgot to eat for hours.

That's what I'm talking about here. The more you can keep your mind engaged at work or with your family, the better off you'll be.

Initially, when you first start fasting, this might mean planning some fun activities to do with your friends or family on the weekend. You don't want to sit around bored with nothing to do on the weekends.

This might cause you to eat simply because you were bored, and you didn't have anything better to do. Remember, you just have to survive for 2-4 weeks until you make it to the other side. It'll be well worth it when you do!

How Much Water Should I Drink Per Day?

The next thing you might be wondering is how much water you should be drinking per day in order to stay hydrated. The standard answer is that you should drink eight, eight-ounce glasses of water throughout the day.

However, this is a blanket answer that doesn't suit individual needs. For example, this would have a 5-foot-1 female drinking the same amount as a 6-foot-4 male.

Their hydration needs would be completely different! There are two things I like to use to judge how much water to drink per day. The first is to go by how you feel.

Essentially, use your own internal thirst mechanism and drink water when you're actually thirsty. Your body will tell you when it needs more water.

When you're hydrated, you won't feel thirsty. Now, this may not be enough if you usually don't drink that much water.

That's why the other thing you need to do is judge your hydration by the color of your urine, like I talked about earlier. If your urine is a yellowish color, then you need to start drinking more water.

On the other hand, if your urine is clear, then you're hydrated and good to go. Doing this will help to keep things simple, and it'll be one less thing that you won't have to worry about tracking and measuring.

What Other Benefits Can I Get from Fasting Besides Weight Loss?

The one major benefit of doing intermittent fasting is that it's an easy way to help you burn fat. However, what are some other results that you can expect to see from doing fasting?

The first benefit is that fasting can improve cognitive brain function, which can help you with improving your concentration. Growing up in school, we were told to eat a big hearty breakfast in order to help us perform our best on a big test.

Think about this though—sometimes after eating a high-carb breakfast, have you ever felt sluggish at work or at school? It's not a coincidence as it turns out.

When we eat a heavy amount of carbs, this makes an amino acid called tryptophan more available to the brain. The tryptophan will then change into serotonin.

Serotonin is a neurotransmitter that is primarily responsible for creating feelings of happiness and comfort. The serotonin will eventually convert into melatonin.

You may have heard of melatonin before because it's a popular nighttime supplement that helps you sleep better. Of course, that may be helpful to you if you're taking it before bed.

However, getting extra melatonin from breakfast isn't something we want in the morning if we're trying to stay awake and focus on something! Therefore, by skipping breakfast, we can help to improve our concentration and productivity at work or school.

Another cool benefit is that fasting may be able to help you recover faster from sickness. Whenever you eat, your body has to focus some of its energy on digesting the food you just ate. Thus, by not eating anything, your body can save some of that energy and focus more of its attention on fighting the illness.

A third plus from fasting is that it will help you save two of your most valuable resources—time and money. Let's say you're eating 5-6 meals a day in an effort to lose weight.

This means that you have to spend more time shopping at the grocery store, preparing those meals, eating those meals, and cleaning up afterwards. That's going to eat up a huge chunk of your time, not to mention the extra money you'll have to spend buying that food.

Compare that to fasting, where you'll only be eating 2-3 meals per day. This involves less prep time, less time at the table eating, and less clean up.

You'll have more time to do whatever you enjoy the most. Not only that, but the extra effort you'll have to go through to eat more meals might make you more likely to quit on your diet plan.

The final benefit I want to talk about in regards to fasting is the fact that it allows you to fly under the radar. You'll still get to enjoy eating large sized meals, and people will start to wonder how it is that you're losing weight while eating these larger meals.

The reality is that you're skipping breakfast and saving those calories for later on, but nobody will see that. This is the way it should be.

You don't want to be that guy who says, "Sorry I can't eat that, I'm on a diet." And as long as you're properly measuring macros and using your 15% junk calories wisely, you shouldn't have to worry about uttering that phrase ever again.

I've Hit a Weight Loss Plateau, and I'm Not Losing Weight Anymore. What Should I Do?

Let's say you've been losing weight steadily, and then all of a sudden, you hit a wall. You've stopped losing weight at the pace you originally were.

What should you do? First, just take a deep breath.

As with any major endeavor in life, there will be obstacles that come up seemingly out of nowhere that must be overcome. You don't want to panic and drastically change your diet plan or anything like that.

Instead, the first thing you need to do is try to figure out why your progress has stalled. Go back and check your food logs, see if you've been doing anything different recently.

Have you been eating more calories than you usually do? If that checks out, then honestly assess how diligent you've been in tracking your calories and macros.

Have you been tracking every calorie that you've been eating and drinking? Have you been tracking it accurately?

Make sure you thoroughly check over the data first; the data, if recorded properly, doesn't lie. If you skip over the data and try to change something else, you could be addressing something that wasn't the problem to begin with.

Once you have thoroughly checked over everything, then you may need to adjust your caloric intake. For example, let's say when you first started, you weighed 250 pounds.

You'd figure out your caloric intake by taking 250, multiplying it by 13, and then subtracting 500 from that number. That would give you a total of 2,750 calories per day in this case.

Now let's say that you've lost 30 pounds and weight loss has stalled. It may be time to update your numbers.

What you'd do now is take your new bodyweight of 220 and multiply it by 13. Then take that number and subtract 500 from it.

This would now give you a total of 2,360 calories per day. If you feel that you're really close to reaching your goal bodyweight, then only subtract 250 from your calculated resting metabolic rate instead of 500.

This will have you losing half a pound a week instead of a pound. You'll also need to recalculate your new protein, carb, and fat intakes as well.

The macro percentages of 40% protein, 35% fat, and 25% carbs will always stay the same regardless of how many calories you're eating per day. Note that you only want to update your caloric needs when progress has halted.

If things are going great and you're losing weight, don't change your numbers. If it isn't broken, then don't try to fix it.

Is It Possible to Change Body Types?

The short answer to that is no, it's not possible to change your body type. If you're a true endomorph, you're not going to be able to transform yourself into an ectomorph.

You're not going to be able to change to a smaller bone structure or develop longer limbs like that of an ectomorph. However, with the proper lifestyle choices such as eating right and exercise, you can start to take on characteristics of another body type.

For example, you might be able to get lean enough to where you start to look more like a mesomorph rather than an endomorph. An ectomorph on the other hand, can build muscle and start to resemble a look more like a mesomorph.

You can also boost your metabolism to more closely resemble that of a mesomorph as well. Will your metabolism ever be as lightning fast as a true ectomorph, or will you burn off carbs as easily as an ectomorph?

Probably not, but that doesn't mean you can't improve your body's ability to use fat for fuel instead of carbs. Conversely, an ectomorph or mesomorph won't be able to match your potential for muscle and strength.

This is all about improving at the end of the day. Take what you've been given and make it better.

You're not in control of your genetics, so instead focus on what you are in control of. Keep in mind that the opposite of this can also be true.

For example, a mesomorph could start to resemble more of an endomorph body type through poor lifestyle choices. Maybe the mesomorph becomes sedentary and eats junk food all of the time.

Then a gut starts to form, and he's starting to look more like an endomorph. Even if someone is born with the awesome genetics of a mesomorph, it doesn't matter.

Regardless of who you are, dedicated effort still has to be put forth in order for you to reach your goals.

Can I Eat Snacks In Between Meals?

I'm not a big fan of snacking, and I haven't been for most of my life. It never made sense to me to eat a little snack that would rarely do anything to keep me full.

If I'm going to eat something, I want it to be a meal that can actually get me full instead of a little snack. Most of the time, snacking is bad for most people.

There are a couple of reasons for this. The first one is that you might not be snacking simply because you're hungry.

You could be snacking because you're bored and you want to distract yourself. Snacking because you're bored isn't a good way to pass the time—it's a good way to take you farther away from your goals!

Having specific times for when you'll eat your regular meals will ensure that you won't engage in mindless eating just because you're bored.

If you find yourself tempted to snack because you're bored, find another way to distract yourself that doesn't involve eating extra calories.

The other reason why I'm not a fan of snacking is that most of the time, the foods you're eating aren't that healthy! Typically, people snack on foods like crackers, chips, cookies, candy, and other junk food.

These simple sugars and starches will provide you with no nutritional value, meaning they're empty calories.

They won't fill you up at all, so you'll still end up eating just as much as you would during your regular meals.

And thanks to the spike in insulin, you'll also get to deal with blood sugar crashes and possible food cravings.

A lot of the time, snacking goes hand-in-hand with convenience. We grab whatever snacks are most accessible.

This will usually involve some sort of pre packaged snack we buy at the store that isn't that healthy for us.

Or maybe we get some junk food from the vending machine during a break at work. The truth is that it's much more difficult to prepare a healthy snack ahead of the time.

Taking the time to prepare a healthier snack that might involve fruit, vegetables, almonds or some protein powder would be much better.

Even with that being the case, it's still better to skip snacks altogether.

Instead, save those calories for later on during your regular meals, and you'll get to enjoy eating more calories. It's that much less food you have to prepare, eat, and clean up, even if it is just a snack.

Conclusion

Thank you so much for reading this book all the way to the end! I hope this book changed the way you view losing weight.

At the end of the day, it all comes down to being able to do what's sustainable, staying diligent, and actually keep up with the plan. I created this endomorph diet in a way that will work with your body type, not against it, in order to help set you up for long-term success.

The rest is up to you. You now have a plan that will be able to guide you to where it is that you want to go; you just have to execute that plan.

Remember that we all have our challenges that we must face and overcome. Weight loss may have been something you've struggled with your whole life, but now you have the right information and the power to change that once and for all.

Yes, there are going to be adversities that you're going to have to overcome. Keep in mind though that there are some benefits to being an endomorph.

You're the strongest of the three body types, and you can build muscle the easiest. That's something ectomorphs wish they had an easier time with.

Focusing purely on your weaknesses and comparing yourself to others is only going to hurt you in the long run. Regardless of what body type you are, don't forget that no one is born with a healthy and fit body that maintains itself by doing nothing and eating junk food.

Whatever fitness goal it is that you want to achieve, you have to be willing to put in the work to be able to achieve it. With that being said, I wish you the best of luck on your fitness journey; I know you can do it!

Did you enjoy reading this book? If so, please consdier leaving a review. Even just a few words would help others decide if the book is right for them.

Best regards and thanks in advance!—Thomas

Sources

(1) https://www.ncbi.nlm.nih.gov/pubmed/22825659

(2)
https://www.ncbi.nlm.nih.gov/pmc/articles/PMC4853817/

(3)
https://www.ncbi.nlm.nih.gov/pmc/articles/PMC5663956/

(4) https://www.ncbi.nlm.nih.gov/pubmed/19860889

(5) https://www.ncbi.nlm.nih.gov/pubmed/18282674

(6) https://www.ncbi.nlm.nih.gov/pubmed/8875519

(7) https://www.ncbi.nlm.nih.gov/pubmed/1765061

(8)
https://www.ncbi.nlm.nih.gov/pmc/articles/PMC3838844/

(9) https://www.mayoclinic.org/healthy-lifestyle/weight-loss/expert-answers/vitamin-b12-injections/faq-20058145

(10)
https://www.ncbi.nlm.nih.gov/pmc/articles/PMC3010674/

(11)
https://www.ncbi.nlm.nih.gov/pmc/articles/PMC2958879/

(12) https://www.ncbi.nlm.nih.gov/pubmed/7369170

(13)
https://www.sciencedirect.com/science/article/pii/S1871403X17300066

(14) https://www.ncbi.nlm.nih.gov/pubmed/7470437